Competency-Based Critical Care

For other titles published in this series, go to
http://www.springer.com/

Mark E. Tomlin (Ed.)

Pharmacology and Pharmacokinetics

A Basic Reader

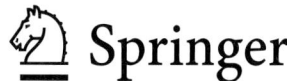

Editor
Mark E. Tomlin, BPharm MSc
Consultant Pharmacist, Critical Care
Department of Pharmacy
Southampton University Hospital
Southampton
UK

ISBN: 978-1-84996-145-5   e-ISBN: 978-1-84996-146-2
DOI: 10.1007/978-1-84996-146-2
Springer Dordrecht Heidelberg London New York

Library of Congress Control Number: 2010925796

Springer is part of Springer Science+Business Media (www.springer.com)

Contents

Contributors

Dr Spike Briggs, BSc, BM, FRCA, CENG
Consultant in Intensive Care Medicine and
   Anesthesia
Poole Hospital NHS Foundation Trust
Poole, UK

David T. Brown BPharm, PhD, MRPharmS
Professor of Pharmacy Practice
School of Pharmacy and Biomedical Sciences
University of Portsmouth
Portsmouth, UK

Dr Mike Celinski, BSc, MBBS, MRCP, FRCA
Consultant in Anesthesia and Intensive Care
Anaesthetic Department
Southampton General Hospital
Southampton, UK

Sue A. Hill, MA, PhD, FRCA
Consultant Anaesthetist
Shackleton Department of Anaesthesia
Southampton General Hospital
Southampton, UK

Dr Kenwyn James, BA(Hons), MBBS, MRCP, FRCA
Consultant, Anesthetics
Southampton University Hospitals NHS Trust
Southampton, UK

Dr Rob Lewis, MBBS, MRCP, FRCA
Consultant in Anasthesia and Intensive Care
Department of Anaesthesia
Ipswich Hospital
Ipswich, UK

Mark E. Tomlin, BPharm, MSc
Consultant Pharmacist, Critical Care
Department of Pharmacy
Southampton University Hospital
Southampton, UK

1
Pharmacology

Sue Hill

Introduction

In this section, we will describe some of the basic principles of how drugs work (pharmacology), how drugs are used (therapeutics) and how drugs are handled by the body (pharmacokinetics). We also need to remember that posology (drug doses) can be fundamental in differentiating between benefits and toxicity.

Mammalian cells consist of a cellular membrane surrounding groups of specialized organelles. It is these sub-cellular organelles that differentiate eukaryotes from prokaryotes like bacteria. The organelles also provide a variety of targets for poisons or drugs. In many cases, the same chemical is poisonous to healthy cells at high doses or produces therapeutic effects at lower doses. Cytotoxic chemotherapeutic agents lack even this distinction and rely on malignant cells that replicate rapidly and accumulate the agent and die before healthy cells suffer excess toxicity. Methotrexate is an antimetabolite cytotoxic drug that binds to the enzyme that activates folic acid in the synthesis of purine bases for DNA. In high doses, healthy human cells need folinic acid (an alternative pathway for purines) to rescue them from excess toxicity.

Antimicrobials differ in their relative accumulation within microbes and mammalian cells. Sometimes, bacteria have different, simpler internal processes that lack alternative pathways for making essential nutrients such as the antifolate antibiotics trimethoprim or sulphonamides. In high doses, the species selectivity may be lost and folic acid may need to be given to avoid bone marrow suppression of the human host.

Within human tissue, drugs often exploit the differences between structures or groups of cells to have therapeutic uses. Blood flow is enhanced when platelets (non-nucleated) cannot synthesize thromboxane, because aspirin has irreversibly blocked the cyclo-oxygenase enzyme when they were formed. However, blood vessel cells (nucleated) can synthesize fresh enzyme and restore prostacyclin production. Thus aspirin has benefits at low doses, but these are diminished or lost as the dose increases.

Unfortunately, as knowledge grows, the pharmacology of drugs appears to change. When I first learnt about sodium nitroprusside, its actions were explained by free cyanide ions poisoning the chain of electron transfer of cytochrome A in respiration. Later, we discovered that this was the toxicity pathway and the benefits came from the release of nitric oxide. Thus keeping up-to-date is essential to maintain safe and evidence-based practice.

Mammalian cells are surrounded by a thin plasma membrane and this is often the site of drug action. Opening the pores in the cell and allowing, loss, gain or exchange of electrolytes or other intracellular components is a primary pharmacological effect. Understanding how this membrane functions is crucial to know whether chemicals will attach to, or pass through, the plasma membrane. The plasma membrane is a complex bipolar layer with an external hydrophilic (water loving) and internal hydrophobic/lipophilic (fat loving) component. Thus chemicals that are highly lipophobic will not bind to the exterior surface of cells unless specific binding sites (or receptors) attract them. Consequently, most drugs are amphiphilic

M. Tomlin (ed.) *Competency-Based Critical Care*,
DOI: 10.1007/978-1-84996-146-2_1, © Springer-Verlag London Limited 2010

loving both water and fat to various degrees, or posses both hydrophilic and hydrophobic centres.

This is why some drugs are difficult to formulate into medicine like injections and require complex co-solvents or solubilizing agents. Mixing drugs can therefore be problematic and the practitioner is advised to be cautious if the medicine is unfamiliar.

Amphotericin is poorly soluble in water (and therefore lipophilic) and the deoxycholate salt is required to get any dissolution (Fungizome). When injected, it is favourably taken up by fungal cells and bound to an internal sterol compound producing a therapeutic benefit in fungaemia. However, the size of the molecule favours scavenging by the reticuloendothelial system and accumulation in the liver. Here it is metabolized and eliminated, but not before causing damage to the liver processing cells. Amphotericin with a fancy liposomal coating (Ambisome) has limited toxicity to the liver. The liposome is phagocytosed by white blood cells on their way to bind to invading fungal cells. The Candida or fungi are then exposed to the pharmacological and toxic effects of amphotericin. The chemical agent is then cleared by different pathways and does not accumulate in the liver. Thus the dose range of Fungizome is 0.25–1 mg/kg and that of Ambisome 1–3 mg/kg.

Mechanism of Drug Action

There are many ways in which drugs bring about their effects. Some drugs are enzyme inhibitors, such as the analgesic non-steroidal anti-inflammatory drugs and some interfere with molecular transport mechanisms, such as the antidepressant serotonin-selective re-uptake inhibitors. Other drugs rely entirely on their physicochemical properties to bring about their effects; a good example is the use of antacid drugs that neutralize the acidic stomach contents. However, many drugs interfere with specific proteins that are essential for signal transduction across membranes or synapses. The next section will focus on this particular mechanism of drug action (Calvey and Williams 2001; Patyrick 2001).

Receptor Interactions

Many drugs act by interacting with receptors, which are large proteins that may be associated with cellular structures, in particular, cell membranes, cytoplasm, intracellular membranes or the nucleus. Binding of a drug to specific and selective sites on receptors then induces a conformational change that is responsible for triggering molecular events that lead to the observed physiological response. Selectivity is due to the 3-dimensional chemical configuration of the drug, which matches the active site on the receptor in a lock and-key fashion; a mechanism similar to the interaction between an enzyme and specific substrates. Initial attraction may be due to ionic forces, but stabilization is due to van der Waals interactions once the drug is in close proximity to its selective binding site.

Cellular receptors may be classified in several ways

- According to the natural ligand, e.g. adrenoceptors, cholinoceptors
- According to the speed of signalling
  - Very fast
  - Moderately fast
  - Slow
- According to the functional type of the receptor
  - Ion channels
  - Transmembrane linked to secondary messenger systems
  - Cytosolic with translocation to the nucleus

The latter system will be used here; in general, ion channels account for very fast responses, transmembrane transduction mechanisms are moderately fast and the cytosol/nuclear type have the slowest onset of action.

Ion Channels

It is important to distinguish ion channels that are opened as a result of changes in membrane potential in the vicinity of an ion channel (voltage-gated channels) from those that are associated with the binding of neurotransmitters (ligand-gated channels). Ligand-gated ion channels are typically found at synapses, associated with both pre- and post-synaptic membranes. Although some voltage-gated ion channels are present pre-synaptically, they are most commonly found in the nerve axon or the non-synaptic regions of the membranes of both the smooth and skeletal muscle.

FIGURE 1.1. Local anaesthetics are weak bases; at body pH, they exist in both ionized and unionized forms, the ratio dependent on their pK_a. The unionized form can more readily pass through the nerve sheath and the cell membrane, but the ionized form is active from within the cell.

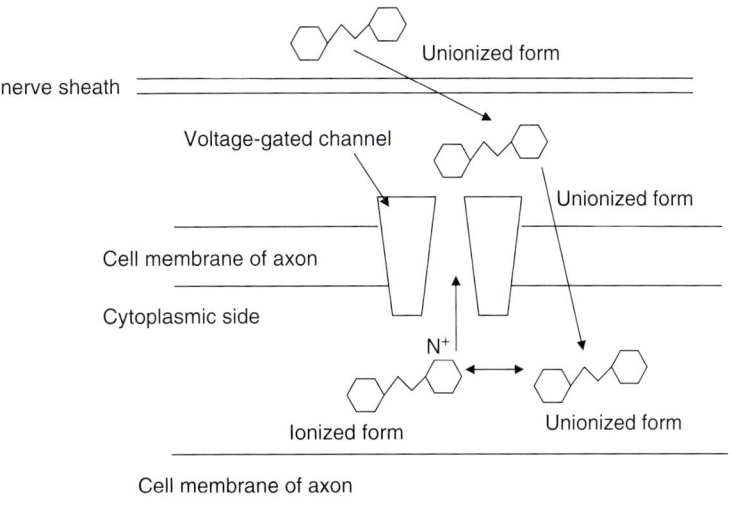

Voltage-Gated Ionic Channels

Local anaesthetics such as lidocaine and bupivacaine act by blocking voltage-gated sodium channels. They are usually administered in close proximity to peripheral neurons; activity requires access to the cytosolic side of the axon, so lipid solubility is important, although the ionized form is active (Figure 1.1). Certain local anaesthetics show use-dependency in that the onset of action is faster if the nerve in question is active, allowing opening of the ion channels. Some anticonvulsants, such as lamotrigine and carbamazepine, act by blockade of central sodium channels thereby reducing neuronal excitability.

Voltage-gated calcium-channel blockers such as nifedipine and verapamil act by blocking L-type calcium channels. The antihypertensive and antianginal effects are associated with the action on vascular smooth muscle, whereas myocardial effects produce their antiarrhythmic action. Central T-type calcium channels are blocked by the anticonvulsant ethosuxamide.

Potassium channels are also blocked by local anaesthetics, although at a higher dose. Voltage-gated potassium channels are blocked by 3,4--diaminopyridine used in the treatment of Lambert–Eaton syndrome, an autoimmune presynaptic disorder of neuromuscular transmission resulting in a myasthenic-type disorder.

Ligand-Gated Ion Channels

These are typified by neurotransmitter-gated ion channels that mediate very rapid transmission of information through the central and peripheral nervous systems. Activation of ligand-gated channels either depolarizes the post-synaptic membrane allowing forward transmission of electrical signals (such as acetylcholine at the motor end-plate) or hyperpolarizes the membrane inhibiting such signals (such as gamma aminobutyric acid, GABA, at GABA type A receptors). There are three distinct families of ligand-gated receptors distinguished by their subunit structure: the pentameric, the ionotropic glutamate and the ionotropic purinergic receptors (Figure 1.2).

Cys-loop pentameric family: e.g. the nicotinic acetylcholine receptor (nACh), the gamma-amino butyric acid type A receptor (GABA$_A$), inhibitory glycine receptors and the 5-hydroxytryptamine (serotonin) type 3 receptor (5HT$_3$).

Each subunit of this pentameric family has four helical transmembrane domains (TMDs) – a domain is a part of a protein chain that plays an important role in the function of that protein, often with a specific 3-D folded shape – none of which is re-entrant (a term used when a protein chain traverses the membrane and loops back on itself without exiting the opposite side of the membrane). The name cys-loop comes from the fact that near the N-terminal, extracellularly, there

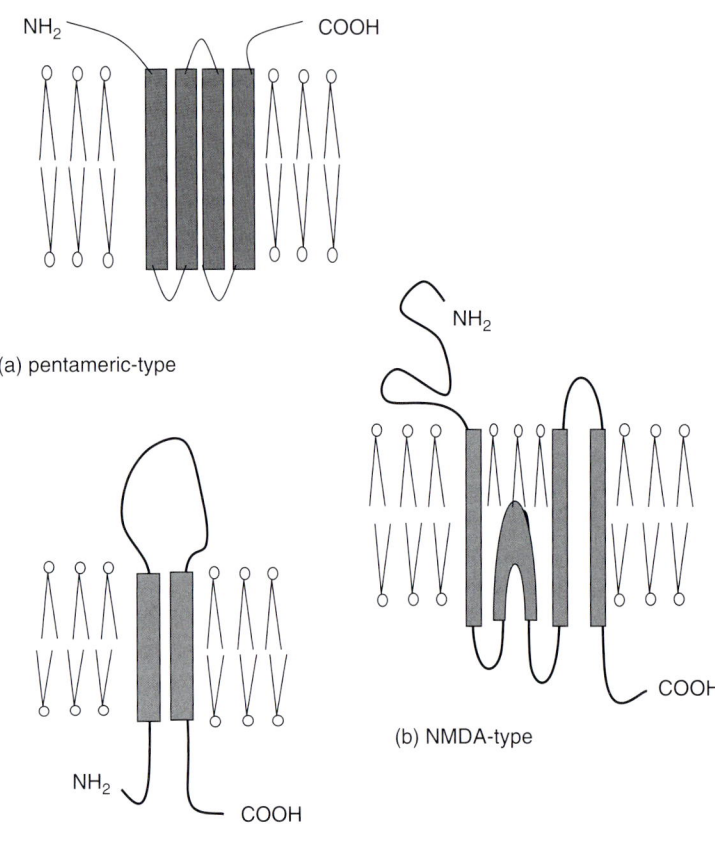

FIGURE **1.2.** Different families of ligand-gated ion channels.

(a) pentameric-type

(b) NMDA-type

(c) purinergic-P2X-type

are two disulphide cysteine bridges, which force the N-terminal into a looped structure.

The pentameric family provides the most important sites of drug action for neuromuscular blocking agents (nACh) and, as has been recognized more recently, for many of our general anaesthetic agents (GABA$_A$); the action of general anaesthetic agents will be discussed in greater detail in Part 2. Subunit composition can vary for the nACh. At the neuromuscular junction (NMJ), the composition is αεαβδ, but in the foetus, it is αγαβδ. Acetylcholine binds to the α–ε and α–δ subunit interfaces, the binding site is formed by at least three peptide loops on the α subunit (principle component) and two on the adjacent subunit (complementary component). Co-operative binding of two molecules of acetylcholine is required to produce the required conformational change and open the channel, which is then five times more selective for monovalent cations – Na$^+$ in particular – than for divalent cations such as Ca^{2+}. Depolarizing neuromuscular blocking agents, such as succinylcholine, bind to the same site

as the natural transmitter acetylcholine and cause opening of the ion channel by inducing conformational changes similar to those induced by acetylcholine, although channel opening time is increased. However, succinylcholine is not rapidly hydrolyzed as it dissociates from the receptor, because it is not a substrate for acetylcholinesterase. As a result, the receptor cannot return to the resting conformation, but becomes desensitized and is no longer able to respond to agonist. This then produces the observed neuromuscular blockade. Acetylcholine alone can also produce blockade, as is seen when acetylcholinesterase is irreversibly inhibited by organophosphates. In contrast, the non-depolarizing muscle relaxants compete for the same binding site as acetylcholine, but the conformational change they induce prevents channel opening. Temporarily increasing the concentration of acetylcholine in the synaptic cleft by the inhibition of acetylcholinesterase will overcome this blockade.

Nicotinic receptors are found at sites other than the NMJ, in particular at autonomic ganglia and in the central nervous system (CNS). In the CNS, the subunit composition is very different from that at the NMJ, $2\alpha3\beta$ or 5β subunits, which accounts for the differing sensitivity of these receptors to cholinergic drugs. In addition, calcium permeability is much greater in CNS nicotinic receptors and they are sensitive to the effects of certain general anaesthetic agents.

The $GABA_A$ and glycine receptors are the major inhibitory signal transducers in the CNS; glycine predominately in spinal cord and hindbrain, GABA supraspinally. The $GABA_A$ channel, unlike the nACh channel, is an anionic channel favouring chloride passage through the synaptic membrane resulting in hyperpolarization and inhibition of forward signalling. Subunit stochiometry depends on anatomical location, but $1\alpha{:}2\beta{:}2\gamma$ and $2\alpha{:}2\beta{:}1\gamma$ are commonly found. The benzodiazepine receptor site is associated with the $GABA_A$ receptor, and is responsible for sedative and anticonvulsant effects due to positive allosteric modulation of the hyperpolarizing signal associated with GABA transmission. The benzodiazepine binding site requires both α- and γ-subunits to be present for positive allosteric modulation whereas etomidate binds with higher affinity to receptors with a β_2 or β_3 subunit.

Ondansetron inhibits 5-hydroxytryptamine type 3 ($5HT_3$) ionotropic channels. Like nACh channels, $5HT_3$ receptors are cation channels favouring monovalent over divalent cations. There are several types of serotoninergic receptors, but only subtype 3 are ionotropic; the others are all G-protein coupled receptors. The centrally mediated anti-emetic action is associated with vagolytic effects as these receptors are also found on vagal afferents from the gastrointestinal tract. Ondansetron therefore has both central and peripheral actions.

Ionotropic Glutamate Receptors

There are three ionotropic (ion-channel associated) glutamate receptor types, NMDA, AMPA and kainate; other glutamate receptors are metabotropic (G-protein coupled). NMDA receptors require co-activation by glycine and glutamate. They are comprised of two subunits, one pore-forming (NR1) and one regulatory, which binds glycine (NR2 A–D types). In vivo, it is thought that the receptors dimerize, forming a complex with four subunits. Each NR1 subunit has three membrane spanning helices, two of which are separated by a re-entrant pore-forming loop that enters and exits the membrane at its cytoplasmic surface. The C-terminus is cytoplasmic, the N-terminus extracellular. All glutamate receptors are equally permeable to Na^+ and K^+, but have a particularly high permeability to the divalent cation, Ca^{2+}, unlike the pentameric excitatory channels. NMDA receptors are of great interest to anaesthetists, because they are the site of action of ketamine, nitrous oxide and xenon, all of which are non-competitive inhibitors of glutamate. There is a high density of NMDA receptors in the hippocampus and associated regions, all of which are important in the formation and recall of memories.

Ionotropic Purinergic Receptors: P2X Subtypes

This family of receptors has two transmembrane domains (TMD) and no pore-forming loops. They form cation channels that are equally permeable to Na^+ and K^+ and also to Ca^{2+}. These receptors are readily inactivated at higher membrane potentials somewhat like voltage-gated Na^+ channels in nerve membranes. They are activated by ATP and its metabolites and are widely distributed in both central and peripheral neurons. The analgesic property of pentobarbital is thought to be due to the inhibition of P2X receptors in the dorsal root ganglia. These ionotropic receptors are not to be confused with G-protein coupled purinergic receptors, i.e. all P1 (adenosine receptors) and P2Y subtypes.

Transmembrane Transducing Receptors

There are several types of transmembrane receptors that trigger secondary messenger effects. The largest group is the G-protein coupled receptors; other types include the tyrosine kinase receptor and the guanyly cyclase-coupled receptor.

G-Protein Coupled Receptors (GPCRs)

Almost 1,000 genes have been identified for GPCRs; many are yet to be characterized. Each GPCR has seven helical TMDs that span the cell membrane, starting with the extracellular N-terminus and ending with the intracellular C-terminus. The quaternary structure is such that these helices cluster together. When a ligand binds, the helices are thought to twist in relation to each other, thereby inducing a large conformational change that is transmitted to the cytoplasmic elements associated with G-protein coupling. The third transmembrane domain, together with the second and third extracellular loops, is specific for a given GPCR and correlates with the ligand binding site. The second and third intracellular loops are associated with G-protein binding. Seven distinct families of GPCRs have been identified; they differ particularly in terms of the relative proximity of the ligand-binding site to the helical domains within the membrane. Compared with other GPCRs, metabotropic glutamate receptors have an extremely large extracellular component. Evidence is accumulating that GPCRs must dimerize (pair up) to form an active complex.

G-Proteins

There are three proteins that associate to form a G-protein, which is associated with the inner leaflet of the lipid bilayer. The type of G-protein is determined by the α-subunit, which has GTPase activity. There are four families of G-protein:

- *Gs* activate adenylyl cyclase to form cAMP
- *Gq* activate β-class phospholipase C polypeptides, especially phospholipase Cβ. As a result, IP_3 (inositol triphosphate) and DAG (di-acyl glycerol) are formed from phosphatidylinositol, a component of cell membranes

- *Gi* family inhibit isoforms of adenylyl cyclase and reduce cAMP
- G_{12} regulate K+ channels

All adrenoceptors, muscarinic, cholinergic and opioid receptors work through a GPCR mechanism. G-proteins are associated with the inner leaflet of the cell membrane and are not normally closely associated with receptors. On binding of the ligand, a conformational change increases the likelihood of the receptor becoming associated with its particular subtype of G-protein(Figure 1.3). The kinetics of GPCR-G-protein interactions requires complex models to explain the observed responses. Essentially, the receptor can exist in a number of states that differ in their affinity for agonist, antagonist or inverse agonist; each of these may or may not be associated with G-protein coupling. Response is greatest when a full agonist is bound to the appropriate G-protein. Once the GPCR-G-protein association takes place, there is a conformational change in the G-protein α subunit that allows GDP to dissociate in exchange for GTP. This in turn allows the α subunit to split away from the βγ dimer. The GTP-bound α subunit now has sufficient energy to interact with intracellular enzymes or cell membrane-bound ion channels and either activate or inhibit these secondary mechanisms. The GTPase activity of the α subunit limits the duration of this activity and once GTP is hydrolyzed to GDP, further interaction is energetically unfavourable and the α subunit then re-associates with the βγ dimer, which has dissociated from the GPCR. In some situations,

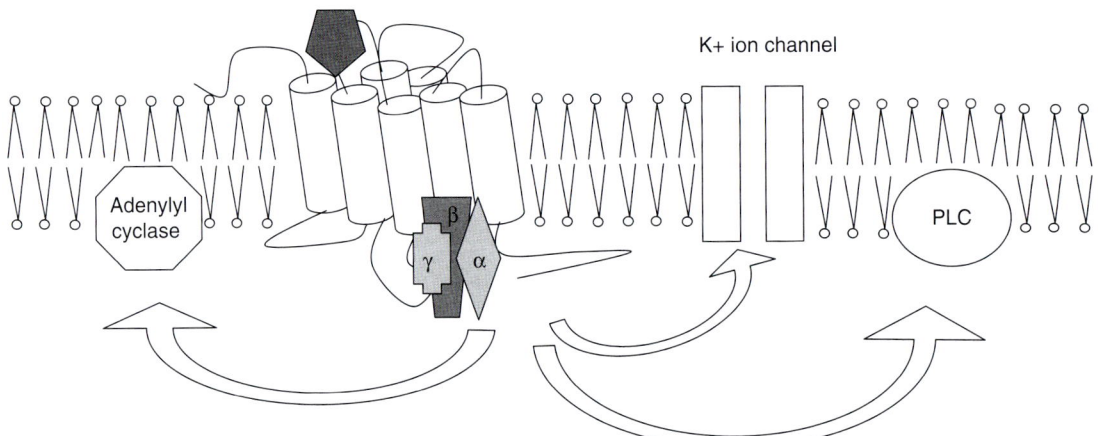

Figure 1.3. G-protein coupled receptors bind a ligand (pentangle) and then activate the appropriate G-protein (trimer shown diagonally opposite the ligand). The G-protein can then affect the function of the enzyme adenylyl cyclase or activate the enzyme phospholipase C (PLC) or may alter ion channel opening.

TABLE 1.1. Some important G-protein coupled receptors and their agonists and antagonists

Natural ligand/receptor type	G-protein α subunit type	Agonist/antagonist drugs
Acetylcholine M1,3,5	Gq	Atropine, glycopyrrolate antagonists
Acetylcholine M2, 4	Gi	Atropine, ipratropium, glycopyrrolate antagonists
Noradrenaline α1	Gq	Phenylephrine agonist; phentolamine antagonist
Noradrenaline α2	Gi	Clonidine agonist; yohimbine antagonist
Noradrenaline β1 and 2	Gs	Isoprenaline, salbutamol agonist (β2); atenolol, propranolol, labetolol antagonist
Opioid receptors (all types)	Gi	Morphine, fentanyl, alfentanil, remifentanil (mu); pentazocine (kappa) agonist
GABA_B receptors	Gi	baclofen agonist
P1 adenosine receptors	Gi	Adenosine agonist
P2Y12 receptors	Gi	ADP agonist; Clopidogrel irreversible antagonist
Histamine H1 receptors	Gq	Cetirizine antagonist
Histamine H2 receptors	Gs	Ranitidine antagonist
Dopamine D1 and D5 receptors (post-synaptic)	Gs	Dopamine and dobutamine in kidney agonist
Dopamine D2–4 receptors (pre-synaptic)	Gi	Bromocriptine agonist; haloperidol, risperidone, chlorpromazine and clozapine (D4 selective) antagonists
Serotonin 5HT1_A receptors	Gi	Buspirone antagonist
Serotonin 5HT2 receptors	Gs	Ketanserin antagonist/inverse agonist
Angiotensin II AT_1 receptors	Gq	Losartan, valsartan antagonist

the βγ dimer can also act as an activator of secondary mechanisms. Examples of drugs acting through this important mechanism are given in Table 1.1.

Tyrosine Kinase Receptors (TKR)

Unlike GPCRs, TKRs do not rely on an intermediary protein for activity, but incorporate the enzyme site on the transmembrane protein itself; the cytoplasmic portion of the receptor is a kinase that is activated by ligand binding to the extracellular portion of the receptor. Insulin receptors are of the TKR type and it is thought that the two receptors must act together (dimerize) in order to elicit a response.

Guanylyl Cyclase Receptors

Transmembrane receptors of this type can activate membrane-bound guanylyl cyclase that produced cGMP from GTP. All the natriuretic peptides act through this mechanism and are responsible for sodium loss through the kidney. Interestingly, these receptors must dimerize for activity. In subarachnoid haemorrhage, the commonly seen salt-losing nephropathy is thought to result from the increased activity of atrial natriuretic peptide.

Intracellular Membrane-Bound Receptors

Intracellular membranes have GPCRs in addition to receptors that respond to secondary messen-gers produced by ligand-GPCR coupling at the cell membrane. Of particular importance is the control of intracellular calcium; in endoplasmic reticulum, the IP_3 (inositol triphosphate) receptor is important. In sarcoplasmic reticulum (SR), the ryanodine receptor in close association with L-type calcium channels, with calmodulin and calcium as modulators, trigger calcium release for excitation-contraction coupling. Dantrolene acts at the ryanodine receptor to inhibit calcium release from the SR; several families with malignant hyperpyrexia have genetic abnormalities associated with the ryanodine receptor.

Cytosolic Receptors

Receptors within the cell can be associated either with the cytosol or with any of the specialized intracellular membranes; of particular importance are receptors associated with the SR that regulate calcium release.

Cytoplasmic Hormone Receptors

Lipid soluble hormones interact with intracellular cytoplasmic receptors. There is a superfamily of such receptors, including those for sex hormones, corticosteroids, thyroxine and vitamin D_3. These receptors act as ligand-regulated transcription factors that bind to DNA and influence the pattern of RNA production by either increasing or inhibiting specific protein production. In the cytoplasm, these receptors are inactive due to the association with inhibitory proteins. Ligand binding produces a conformational change that activates the receptor and initiates translation to the nucleus and association with specific DNA promotor sequences. Gene transcription is influenced by the recruitment of additional proteins that act as co-activators or co-repressors that remodel the quaternary structure of DNA. Chromatin structure may be loosened, thereby encouraging transcription, or chromatin condensation may be favoured, inhibiting transcription. The oestrogen receptor modulator tamoxifen inhibits transcription associated with tumour cells in certain cancers. In addition to hormone receptors, other nuclear receptors can also influence protein production; the new antidiabetic drug rosiglitazone is a peroxisome proliferator-activated receptor type γ (PPAR-γ) agonist that stimulates protein transcription leading to insulin sensitizing activity within the adipose tissue.

Adrenosteroid Hormones

There are two types of corticosteroid receptor; MR (or type 1) is the mineralocorticoid receptor and GR (or type 2), the glucocorticoid receptor. MR and GR receptors are each composed of four distinct protein regions, including an N-terminal region associated with the activation of transcription, a DNA-binding domain, a nuclear localization signal and a C-terminal hormone-binding region. Glucocorticoid binding displaces the inhibitory heat-shock proteins and triggers a conformational change that facilitates translocation and binding to specific regions on DNA. The GR receptor is widespread in cells, whereas MR is restricted to epithelial tissue such as renal collecting tubules. Cortisol and aldosterone are equipotent at MR receptors; aldosterone-triggered activation is permitted by the presence of 11-β hydroxysteroid dehydrogenase in epithelial cells, which metabolizes cortisol to a compound that is inactive at the MR receptor.

Pharmacodynamics

Introduction to Drug–Receptor Interaction

Binding of a drug to a receptor brings about a response; the magnitude of the response is related to the concentration of the drug–receptor complex that is formed. The assumption that the response is linearly related to the concentration of occupied receptors is then made:

$$\text{Response} = \text{constant (DR)}$$

This applies the law of "mass action" to the binding of a drug to a receptor.

$$D + R \leftrightarrow DR \rightarrow \rightarrow \rightarrow \text{Response}$$

This leads to an equation relating the rates of the forward and reverse reactions at equilibrium:

$$[D] \cdot [R] \cdot k_f = [DR] \cdot k_b$$

where k_f and k_b are the rate constants for the forward and reverse reactions, respectively

Algebraic re-arrangement then gives us:

$$k_b / k_f = K_d = [D] \times [R] / [DR]$$

where K_d is the dissociation constant

We do not know [R], the concentration of unoccupied receptors, but we know that there is a limited number of receptors. If R_t is the total number of receptors then $[R] = [R_t] - [DR]$. Substituting this into the equation above gives:

$$K_d = [D] \cdot ([R_t] - [DR]) / [DR]$$

Algebraic re-arrangement gives:

$$[DR] / [R_t] = \text{fractional occupation}$$
$$(f) = [D] / ([D] + K_d)$$

Since fractional occupation (f) represents response for agonist drugs, a plot of response against concentration of a drug ([D]) will be hyperbolic. When $[D] = K_d$, then $f = 1/2$, i.e. 50% response when the drug concentration is equal to the dissociation constant (Figure 1.4a). In clinical terms, this is generally known as the ED$_{50}$ (the effective dose to produce 50% response). This graph is not ideal for determining K_d or ED$_{50}$. A better graph is that of fractional response against log([D]) – a semi-logarithmic transformation. The resultant curve is sigmoid, with an almost-linear central region, allowing for better comparison of ED$_{50}$ for different agonists in the system (Figure 1.4b).

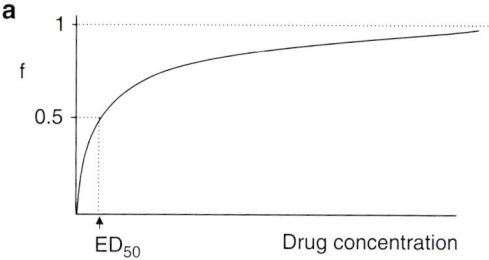

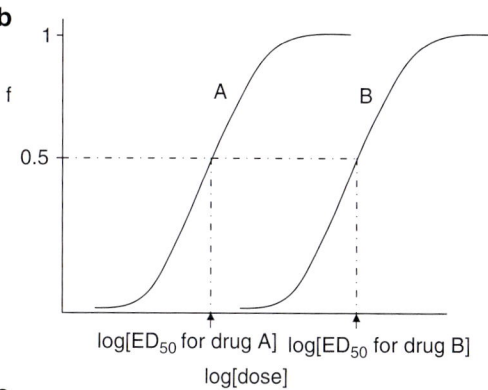

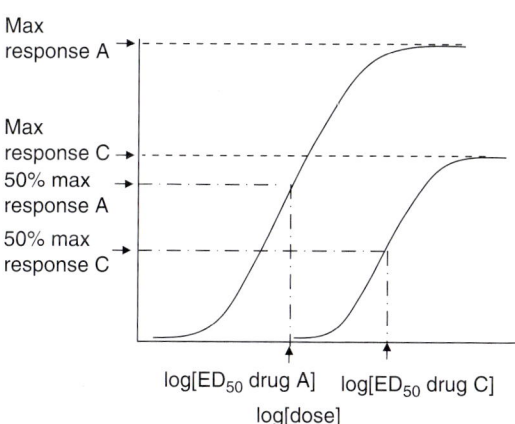

FIGURE 1.4. (**a**) Dose vs. fractional response curve, a rectangular hyperbola; (**b**) log[dose] vs. response curve, a sigmoid shape. In this case, drug A is more potent than drug B as its ED$_{50}$ is lower; (**c**) In this log[dose] vs. response curve, drug A can elicit a maximum response, whereas drug C has a maximum response that is much less than that of drug A. Drug C is a partial agonist, drug A is a full agonist. In addition, drug A is more potent than drug C as it has a lower ED$_{50}$.

Properties of Receptor Systems

Drug–receptor interactions have two important properties: potency and efficacy (sometimes called intrinsic activity). Potency is related to

affinity; drugs with a high affinity have a dissociation constant (K_d) that is low (in the micromolar range) as is their ED$_{50}$. Efficacy or intrinsic activity is related to the maximum possible response for any given system.

Affinity: the tenacity with which the drug binds to the receptor

Efficacy: the capacity of a drug to produce a response once bound to the receptor

- *Full agonists*: efficacy = 1
- *Partial agonists*: 0 < efficacy < 1
- *Competitive antagonists*: efficacy = 0
- *Inverse agonists*: −1 < efficacy < 0

Full agonists have an efficacy of 1, whereas partial agonists have an efficacy that is less than 1 but greater than zero (Figure 1.4c). Antagonists have an efficacy of 0, since they have no effect in the absence of agonist.

Types of Drug–Receptor Interaction

Drugs may act as agonists, antagonists or allosteric modulators.

Types of Agonist

Full Agonist

Drugs that are capable of eliciting the maximum possible response in a system are known as full agonists. Many drugs in use in the ICU are full agonists, e.g. noradrenaline at α-adrenoceptors, morphine at μ-opioid receptors and midazolam at the benzodiazepine receptor.

Partial Agonist

A partial agonist binds to the same site on the receptor as the agonist, but fails to elicit a maximum response, whatever dose of the drug is used. There are relatively few clinically useful drugs that are partial agonists. Buprenorphine is a potent partial agonist at μ-opioid receptors. The reason for their limited use, especially on an ICU, is that if the maximum effect of a partial agonist is insufficient and a full agonist is subsequently added, the partial agonist can act as a competitive antagonist and higher doses of the full agonist will be needed to produce the maximum response. Some β-adrenergic blockers (e.g. practolol and pindolol) have minimal partial agonist properties, which were thought to limit the extent of the resultant bradycardia.

Inverse Agonists

An inverse agonist binds to the same site as the agonist, but elicits the opposite effect. The concept of inverse agonism was first described for the benzodiazepine receptor site, where beta-CCE is an inverse agonist. Some data suggest that flumazanil may have a degree of inverse agonist activity to account for excitatory phenomena associated with high doses, although this is not firmly established. Ketanserin is possibly an inverse agonist at serotonin type 2A receptors. It has been shown that many of our so-called competitive antagonists also possess some inverse agonist action, although their principle use is to antagonize the effects of endogenous agonists (see below).

Types of Antagonist

Antagonists may be reversible or irreversible. Many animal and plant toxins are irreversible inhibitors of neurotransmitter receptors, for example, the snake venom α-bungarotoxin blocks the nicotinic cholinergic receptor at the NMJ.

There are two types of reversible antagonists: competitive and non-competitive.

Competitive Antagonist

These drugs bind to the same site as agonist producing a parallel shift of the log(dose)–response curve (Figure 1.5a). Thus the apparent potency of the agonist is reduced, but the efficacy remains unchanged. The extent of the shift is the log(dose ratio), which is determined by the inhibitor dose and dissociation constant (K_i). If dose ratios are found for different doses of a given antagonist, a

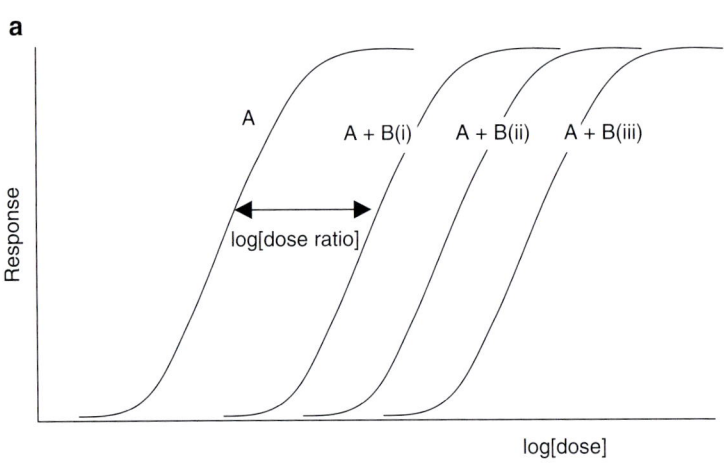

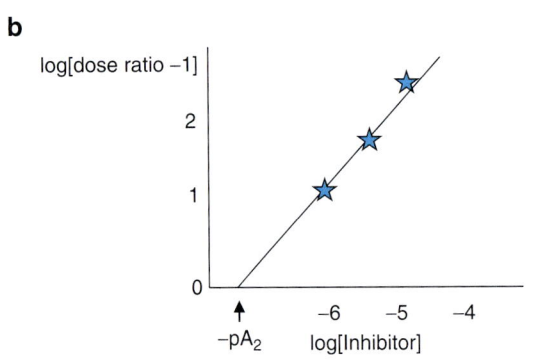

FIGURE 1.5. Competitive inhibition. (**a**) The line A represents agonist alone; lines A + B (i), A + B (ii) and A + B (iii) show the log[dose of agonist] vs. response curve shifting more and more to the right with increasing dose of competitive antagonist present. The extent of the shift is [log (D′)−log(D)], where D and D′ are the agonist doses that produce an equivalent response in the absence and presence of the inhibitor respectively; this is equivalent to log (D′/D) or log(dose ratio). (**b**) A Shild plot. It can be shown that DR = 1 + [I]/K_i so (DR−1) = [I]/K_i, thus log(DR−1) = log([I])−log(K_i). So when the DR is 2, log(DR−1) = log(1) = 0, so log([I])−log(K_i) = 0 and log([I]) = log(K_i). Thus the intercept on the x-axis when log(DR−1) = 0 is log(K_i) = −pA$_2$. (DR: dose ratio; I: concentration of inhibitor; K_i: dissociation constant for the inhibitior).

FIGURE 1.6. Non-competitive antagonism. The efficacy of the agonist is reduced, but the potency is unchanged.

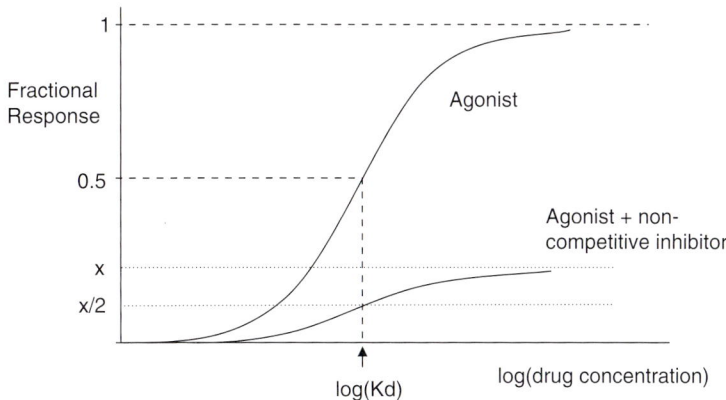

Schild plot (Figure 1.5b) can be used to find pA_2 and K_i. The pA_2 is the negative logarithm of the dose of antagonist that requires a doubling of agonist dose to produce the same response as in the absence of antagonist. It is actually the negative logarithm of the dissociation constant for the inhibitor. Competitive inhibitors encountered in the ICU include non-depolarizing neuromuscular blocking agents such as vecuronium, atracurium and cisatracurium, which inhibit the action of the natural transmitter acetylcholine at the NMJ.

Non-competitive Antagonist

In classical receptor pharmacology, a non-competitive antagonist binds to a different site on the receptor from the agonist site, but does not affect agonist binding, so K_d is the same. However, its presence reduces the maximum possible effect. Thus the slope rather than the position of the curve is changed (Figure 1.6). It has now become more common to use the term non-competitive for any drug that reduces the effectiveness of an agonist by binding to a different site. In this more general definition, both slope and maximum effect can be affected. Thus both classical non-competitive inhibitors and negative allosteric modulators (see below) are generally referred to as non-competitive inhibitors. An example of non-competitive inhibition is the action of ketamine at the NMDA receptor, where the agonist is glutamate.

Allosteric Modulators

Some drugs can alter the effect of an agonist by altering the link between agonist binding and conformational change. The change may either enhance the response (positive allosteric modulation) or reduce the response (negative allosteric modulation). The drug does not bind to the same site as the agonist, but influences the affinity of agonist for the receptor as well as the efficacy. Benzodiazepines are positive allosteric modulators at the GABA type A receptors in the central nervous system. These are inhibitory receptors that, when activated hyperpolarize and reduce the responsiveness of the post-synaptic membrane. They are thought to be involved in producing hypnosis and anaesthesia. Propofol and thiopentone can act as positive allosteric modulators at this receptor, but through a different binding site than benzodiazepines.

References

Calvey TN, Williams NE (eds) (2001) Drug action. In: Principles and practice of pharmacology for anaesthetists, chap. 3, 4th edn. Blackwell Science, Oxford. ISBN: 0-632-05603-3

Patrick GL (ed) (2001) The why and the wherefore. In: An introduction to medicinal chemistry, chap. 2, 2nd edn; Oxford University Press, Oxford. ISBN: 0-19-850533

2
Pharmacokinetic Principles

David Brown and Mark Tomlin

Introduction

In general medicine, we give a drug to a patient at a recommended dose and anticipate a therapeutic response. Most Phase 3 clinical trials produce data that tell us what a ballpark dose should be for an average patient to achieve a usual effect, and if we are lucky, what to expect in terms of side effects at usual doses or if doses are exceeded.

We are sometimes surprised when the usual dose either fails to elicit any kind of response or produces side effects that, according to our evidence, should be observed only at much higher doses.

Most drug effects are achieved by the interaction of a drug with receptors on the target organ. The intensity and duration of that effect are usually determined by the number of drug molecules present, their receptor site binding affinity, and their residence time at the receptor site(s). This *pharmacodynamic* aspect of drug therapy is discussed in detail in Chapter 1.

After administration, by whatever route, the drug concentration at the target site is governed by the often tortuous route its takes to get there. Like any journey, it can be planned in terms of route directions, load, and time, and calculations can be used to show what load can be delivered at a particular speed over what terrain, and what hazards must be overcome to reach the destination successfully. This road map is the essence of *pharmacokinetics* – the study of time-dependent drug movement into, around and out of the body.

In a healthy population, there is a natural variation in the pharmacokinetic processes of absorption, distribution, metabolism, and excretion; that is why, average doses will produce average responses, and for many drugs with wide safety margins, this is sufficient. However, some drugs do not have wide safety margins and knowledge of clinical pharmacokinetics in the individual is vital to ensure that therapy with these drugs is effective and as safe as possible. It is also important to recognize that organ disease, particularly that of the liver and kidney, can affect pharmacokinetics profoundly and patients with such comorbidities should be monitored appropriately. Nowhere is this more important than in critical care where patient status may change rapidly with time, requiring a thorough knowledge of pharmacokinetics. To use the above analogy, the road map may be poorly defined, particularly for new drugs, and subject to frequent and sometimes misleading updates along the way.

The following sections summarize the important aspects of pharmacokinetic first principles under the traditional headings of drug absorption, distribution, metabolism, and excretion. With their training in drug structure and action and knowledge of available formulations, pharmacists are in an excellent position to work with anesthetists in this area. As you will see, number crunching to arrive at a suitable solution to individualizing drug therapy is not always a prerequisite, but common sense and the ability to imagine what is happening to the drug inside the patient in front of you are.

M. Tomlin (ed.) *Competency-Based Critical Care,*
DOI: 10.1007/978-1-84996-146-2_2, © Springer-Verlag London Limited 2010

Drug Absorption

Drug absorption is a prerequisite for drug action. Drugs may have to be absorbed across a number of membranes before they reach the general circulation, depending on the route of administration. Even if they are administered parenterally, any route other than the intravenous one will require subsequent movement from the injection site to the general circulation unless a local effect is required, e.g., intraarticular injection.

Drug absorption may require movement of the drug across barriers as diverse as the mucosal epithelium of the gastrointestinal (GI) tract, which stretches from the sublingual area to the rectum, the lung, external eye structures such as the conjunctiva and the skin, and the vagina. While these outer defenses have a variety of structures, some basic principles may be applied when it comes to the absorption of drugs.

There are two main ways of crossing these barriers that are most relevant to clinical pharmacokinetics:

- Diffusing through the lipid
- Attaching to membrane transport molecules (MTMs) that carry them across

Lipid diffusion

Fick's law of transmembrane diffusion states that the rate of movement of the solute is described by the concentration gradient and the permeability of the barrier (membrane). Large concentration gradients produce faster mass transfer than smaller ones.

Lipid diffusion is passive and driven from an area of high concentration, e.g., the stomach contents where the drug has just been released from a capsule by dissolution, to an area of lower concentration – the enteric circulation. Lipid solubility is one of the most important determinants of drug absorption and subsequent distribution when crossing endothelia such as the blood-brain barrier (BBB) or the placenta. A rule of thumb is that drugs with a high lipid (or oil)/water partition coefficients are absorbed and distributed more rapidly and completely than drugs with lower coefficients. The partition coefficient (P) is determined in vitro and represents the ratio of drug concentrations in the oil (usually octanol) and aqueous phases of a mixture at equilibrium. It is common to use the log P value for comparative purposes; drugs with log P values increasingly greater than zero (e.g., amiodarone – 1.3; pentobarbital – 2.0; diazepam – 2.7) have increasingly favorable absorption characteristics, while sub-zero values (e.g., gentamicin, vancomycin, ceftriaxone, heparin, and streptokinase) are associated with poorer absorption and distribution into lipid-containing tissues.

Another rule of thumb is that unionized drug molecules are more lipid soluble than their corresponding ionized species; consequently, their absorption is also more rapid and complete. Membrane permeability of normally ionized drugs may be increased by suppressing ionization; either by manipulation of the surrounding pH or by chemical modification to neutralize ionizable groups, for example, by esterification. The potential for ionization in relation to pH is determined by the pK_a, which is the pH at which the compound is 50% ionized. Hence at a gastric pH of 2, aspirin, a weak acid with a pK_a of 3.5, is largely in its unionized form and a significant amount is absorbed in the stomach. Although more is ionized in the less-acid environment of the small intestine, a greater quantity is absorbed there due to the relatively large surface area available for absorption. An increase in gastric pH increases gastric emptying rate, which may explain why aspirin absorption increases when given with an antacid!

Pethidine, on the other hand, is a weak base with a pK_a of 8.6 and is largely protonated (ionized) in the stomach. Significant absorption does not take place until the drug reaches the less-acid environment of the small intestine.

Exceptions are gentamicin and vancomycin; they are a polycationic, but even the unionized species are insufficiently lipid soluble to traverse a lipid barrier. These molecules also contain sugar residues that can take part in hydrogen bonding, rendering them too hydrophilic. They have to be given parenterally for a systemic effect and do not cross the BBB or placenta, or penetrate vitreous humor.

There may be other components of the barrier that are important to the successful (or otherwise) passage of drugs. Blood flow on the other side of the membrane may play an important role in maintaining a concentration gradient of sufficient magnitude to drive absorption; if the blood flow is diminished, for example, in congestive heart failure, then the gradient will diminish and absorption will be slowed down. The membrane may also contain metabolic enzymes that destroy the drug in transit leading to reduced bioavailability.

Membrane Transport Molecules

Many biological membranes have transport mechanisms geared to ensuring the safe passage of naturally occurring molecules such as sugars, neurotransmitters, ions, and amino acids. Such systems usually consist of one or more proteins capable of binding the target molecule and promoting transport across the membrane. Some are sufficiently nonspecific to permit drug transport. For example, L-dopa, gabapentin, 5-fluorouracil, and baclofen are transported by attaching to amino acid transporters, and beta-lactams are transported by molecules designed to transport naturally occurring oligopeptides (Shargel et al. 2005).

MTMs work in several different ways: first, by *facilitated diffusion*: no energy is required for the MTM to facilitate the passage of the drug with the existing concentration gradient. Second, by *active transport*: when the drug is transported against the prevailing concentration gradient; this latter process consumes energy. Membrane transport systems are capable of saturation, and a further increase in drug concentration does not result in a further increase in absorption, unless simple lipid diffusion is also occurring. These systems are also prone to competitive inhibition by a second drug or ligand. This phenomenon is exploited in psychopharmacology, where the accumulation of specific neurotransmitters via membrane transport into nerve terminals can be inhibited by specific drugs, exemplified by the selective serotonin reuptake inhibitors.

Several features of MTMs are important from a pharmacokinetic viewpoint. They are capable of saturation, susceptible to competition, and are prone to genetic polymorphism. Significant membrane carrier mechanisms exist in the GI tract, the renal tubules, the biliary tract, and the BBB.

P-Glycoprotein

P-glycoprotein (PGP) is a specific example of a molecule capable of facilitating transmembrane molecular transport. In vitro and in vivo studies have shown that PGP plays an important part in the absorption, distribution, and elimination of many drugs by molecular transfer (Lin 2003). In the gut, PGP acts to exclude foreign molecules, and as such, plays an important role in preventing the entry of foreign, potentially harmful substances. PGP is particularly good at removing lipid-soluble drugs that enter by passive diffusion such as ciclosporin and vinblastine, but vitamin B12, L-dopa and 5-fluorouracil, paclitaxel, and digoxin are also affected. The small intestine is particularly rich in PGP, and by inference, it will exert its greatest effects there, although its inhibiting effect on the passage of some drugs into urine and across the BBB has also been shown (Evans and McLeod 2003). There is a good inverse correlation between duodenal PGP expression and digoxin plasma levels (Hoffmeyer et al. 2000) and evidence that at least one other substrate for PGP, the protease inhibitor ritonavir, may cause competitive inhibition resulting in increased digoxin bioavailability (Phillips et al. 2003).

Like the hepatic microsomal enzyme system, PGP is vulnerable to inhibition, activation, or induction by drugs. The herbal preparation St John's wort induces the intestinal expression of PGP in vitro and in vivo (Hennessy et al. 2002; Izzo 2005) and has been implicated in the reduced bioavailability of HIV protease inhibitors, warfarin, (and digoxin). The absorption of simvastatin, verapamil, tacrolimus, ritonavir, and indinavir is also known to be affected by PGP, but the clinical importance of any PGP-mediated drug interactions is unknown.

For some drugs, interaction with PGP seems inextricably linked to hepatic metabolism. For example, intestinal PGP is inhibited by ciclosporin, resulting in increased bioavailability of both paclitaxel and docetaxel (Terwgot et al. 1999; Malingre et al. 2001); however, ciclosporin also inhibits the hepatic microsomal enzyme CYP3A4 for which paclitaxel and docetaxel are substrates, thus reducing hepatic clearance. It is difficult to dissociate the two effects. Certainly, the observed increase in bioavailability of these two taxanes cannot be explained by PGP inhibition alone.

Lin (2003) has suggested that the observed inter and intra-individual variability in intestinal PGP expression has much to do with the variation in oral absorption of drugs that are PGP substrates. Up to an eightfold variation in PGP expression has been shown in healthy individuals (Lown et al. 1997).

The impact of PGP on drug absorption may, in many cases, be of minor quantitative importance compared to its impact on distribution, such as brain penetration. Just because a drug is a good PGP substrate does not mean that absorption will be poor. Digoxin is a good example. PGP is known to be saturable at relatively low digoxin concentrations in the intestinal lumen and oral bioavailability remains high, probably because passive diffusion predominates.

Other Factors Affecting Drug Absorption

The pH of the delivery compartment can influence dissolution from solid dosage forms, e.g., sodium bicarbonate increases gastric pH and decreases tetracycline dissolution and hence its absorption. Increasing gastric pH will decrease the ionization of weak bases and promote absorption while the reverse is true for weak acids.

Reduced GI blood flow due to congestive heart disease and nephrotic syndrome can reduce the absorption of a range of drugs.

GI transit time is decreased in diarrhea, but increased by immobility; it is also influenced by a number of drugs acting on the mesenteric plexus. The GI transit time can alter both the rate and extent of drug absorption after oral administration. Absorption of an acidic drug such as aspirin is promoted by drugs that accelerate gastric emptying (e.g., metoclopramide) and slowed by drugs that slow emptying, e.g., antimuscarinic agents and narcotic analgesics, in spite of the fact that the acidic environment of the stomach favors the absorption of weak acids. GI hurry may decrease the absorption of drugs with intrinsically slow dissolution rates such as digoxin and specialized formulations such as sustained release and enteric-coated preparations. A practical example of how GI motility can be manipulated is the combination of the antiemetic metoclopramide with paracetamol to optimize analgesic absorption in patients with migraine-associated nausea and vomiting.

Drug metabolizing enzymes, notably CYP3A4, are present in the duodenal, jejunal, and ileal membranes. As with their liver counterparts, expression is subject to genetic polymorphism, induction, competition, and saturation, which all contribute to the variability in response to substrate drugs.

Concomitant membrane disease can affect drug absorption. Most of the interesting examples are to be found in the GI tract. For example, Crohn's disease increases the absorption of clindamycin and propranolol, possibly due to the presence of an inflamed and more easily breached mucosa, but the absorption of most drugs is reduced, notably analgesics and antibiotics. Coeliac disease has a similar effect, causing drug that would normally be absorbed efficiently in the small intestine to be absorbed further down the GI tract where the absorptive environment is less favorable and absorption less complete. Drug absorption will improve with successful treatment of the disease.

The presence of food increases absorption of propranolol, metoprolol, digoxin, and griseofulvin, probably by increasing portal hepatic blood flow. Effects are variable and drug-specific; for example, food increases the absorption of metoprolol by 50%, but decreases absorption of aspirin, penicillins G and V, and atenolol by up to 50%, probably by diluting or complexing with these sparingly lipid-soluble drugs. Some foodstuffs, notably grapefruit juice, inhibit drug metabolizing enzyme in the gut wall, thereby increasing the bioavailability of calcium channel blockers and some statins. Enteral feeds can impair the absorption of highly protein-bound drugs when coadministered; this phenomenon is well-documented with phenytoin (Stockley 2002).

Enteric bacteria can metabolize some drugs such as lactulose (when used to treat hepatic encephalopathy) and oral contraceptive conjugates. Thus gut sterilization can disturb the status quo leading to therapeutic failure.

Coadministered drugs. Gastric emptying may be slowed by atropine, tricyclic antidepressants, or opiates, thus slowing absorption in the duodenum. Absorption may be enhanced by drugs hastening emptying, e.g., metoclopramide and erythromycin. The mucosal protectant sucralfate, which forms a viscous gel covering the mucosal surface, presents an additional barrier to absorption for several important drugs such as theophylline, digoxin, and fluoroquinolone antibiotics.

Drug Absorption from the Lung

The absorption of most anesthetic gases through the lung epithelium is very rapid. Sparingly, lipid-soluble gases (e.g., nitrous oxide) are perfusion limited and absorption depends on the rate of blood flow to maintain a concentration gradient and hence minimize anesthetic concentration. More lipid-soluble gases such as isoflurane are concentration limited; the rate of gas delivery determines absorption. Drug from aerosols intended to produce local effects may be absorbed in appreciable quantities if use is excessively prolonged, dosing is excessive, or mucosal inflammation has occurred. For example, tremor, tachycardia, and hypokalemia have been observed after high dose, nebulized salbutamol.

Drug Absorption Through the Skin

Critical care considerations include the use of fentanyl. The molecule is very lipid soluble and penetrates skin easily. Patch technology assures a constant rate of delivery for a set period for a given dose, but accumulation to effective levels is slow (up to 24 h) and previous analgesia should be phased out gradually to account for this. Similarly, when discontinuing patch therapy, it should be appreciated that decline in fentanyl levels is slow (it may take 17 h for plasma levels to decrease by 50%). Hence, it is important to know if a patient has been using fentanyl prior to transfer to, or from, critical care; replacement opioid therapy should be commenced at low dose and titrated upward to avoid respiratory depression.

Glyceryl trinitrate is another small, lipid-soluble molecule that penetrates skin efficiently. In addition to its use in patch formulations to control angina, it can be used to achieve a local benefit in the prophylaxis of phlebitis and extravasation by applying the patch distal to the site of intravenous cannulation at the time of venepuncture.

IM and SC Absorption

For many drugs, absorption after IM administration is unreliable. Lipid-soluble drugs have better and more predictable absorption because they diffuse better through adipose tissue and capillary walls to reach the general circulation. Less lipid-soluble drugs may be taken up by the lymphatic system. The drug must stay in solution at muscle pH or microcrystallization will occur, release will be delayed, and absorption after redissolution may be unpredictable, e.g., with phenytoin, digoxin, and diazepam. If crystallization is controlled, the phenomenon can be put to good advantage. For example, insulin glargine is formulated at an acid pH; when injected, the drug forms a microprecipitate from which release is prolonged but relatively constant. Midazolam is supplied in solution for IV or IM injection formulated at a pH of less than 4. The imidazo ring remains open in this pH range and the compound is water soluble (see Figure. 2.1). Upon injection, increase to physiological pH promotes closure of the imidazole ring that is accompanied by an increase in lipid solubility, good absorption from an IM site, and subsequent penetration of the BBB.

The rate and extent of absorption depend on muscle blood flow and the amount of fat surrounding the muscle. Sudden exercise can increase body temperature and blood flow and increase drug absorption (e.g., insulin). Subcutaneous

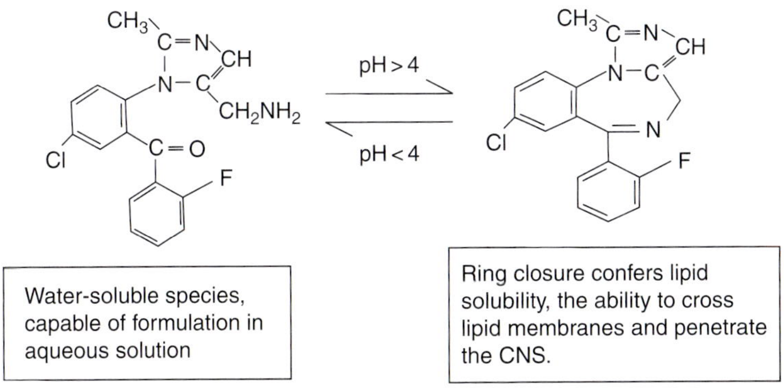

Water-soluble species, capable of formulation in aqueous solution

Ring closure confers lipid solubility, the ability to cross lipid membranes and penetrate the CNS.

FIGURE 2.1. pH-dependent structural changes of midazolam.

injections have similar problems to IM ones. In general, the blood supply is poorer and absorption will be relatively slower.

Bioavailability

One cannot leave the topic of drug absorption without mentioning bioavailability. Essentially, this term is used to describe the amount of drug reaching the general circulation from the delivery system being used. The bioavailability of a drug administered by the intravenous route is 100%. At the other extreme, the bioavailability of a drug given by an inappropriate route (e.g., insulin, erythropoietin, sucralfate, vancomycin, administered by mouth) will be negligible due to its destruction by enzymes, acid hydrolysis, or complexation with stomach contents.

For most drugs, bioavailability falls between these two extremes and is linked to, but not determined exclusively by, lipid solubility. Other factors include its formulation; the physicochemical properties of the drug; its susceptibility to gastric acid and digestive enzymes; the coadministration of other drugs; the presence of comorbidity affecting absorption sites such as diarrhea, vomiting, or malabsorption syndromes; and the degree of metabolism that occurs either in the gut mucosa itself or in the first pass through the liver. For example, the oral bioavailability of cimetidine is 60%, but that of buspirone is only 4% because the latter undergoes extensive "first-pass" metabolism (see below) before it reaches the systemic circulation. Drugs that undergo high first-pass metabolism such as morphine, propranolol, and verapamil have much higher oral than IV doses as a consequence. Drugs with low first-pass metabolism, such as theophylline, phenytoin, and diazepam, have similar oral and IV dosing schedules. The doses for oral, rectal, and IV paracetamol are similar but note variability (20–80% absorption). Even for drugs not subject to first-pass metabolism, the intrinsic absorbability by the oral route may be low. For example, only 40–50% of an oral dose of atenolol is absorbed compared to 100% delivery by the IV route. In addition first pass effects produce an oral dose that is 10 times that of the IV.

In addition to the parenteral routes mentioned above, sublingual and rectal routes allow drugs to avoid first-pass metabolism. Suitable candidates will depend on their physicochemical properties and individual formulation characteristics. For example,

greater than 90% of a single oral or sublingual dose of nifedipine is absorbed and drug appears in serum 10 min after sublingual and 20 min after oral dosing with maximal equivalent serum concentrations being achieved at 1–2 h. These correspond to the equivalent concentrations over the same time period after intravenous administration.

We have already mentioned that formulation can alter the bioavailability of a drug. This is particularly true of medicines that are administered orally. Differences in compaction pressure of tablets, particle size distribution of capsule ingredients, and interactions with other excipients can profoundly alter bioavailability. These parameters are carefully controlled between batch runs for all licensed medicines in the UK, so that variations are minimized; this is particularly important for drugs with narrow therapeutic windows such as digoxin, phenytoin, and theophylline, but variations do exist between different formulations of the same drug. For example, the fraction of digoxin that is "bioavailable" from tablets, liquid, and injection is commonly taken as 70, 80, and 100%, respectively (Winter 2003). This discrepancy is often referred to as the bioavailability factor F, which must be considered when calculating doses delivered from these three formulations. A similar situation exists with sodium fusidate where recommended adult doses for the suspension are 50% higher than those for the tablet formulation.

For true bioequivalence to exist between two products, or even batches of the same product, both the rate and extent of absorption (F) should be identical. In practice, limits are set, relating to the rate of rise of the serum level – time curve to maximum serum concentration (C_{max}), the time taken to achieve this (T_{max}), and the area circumscribed by the curve. If these are exceeded for one product compared to another, the two products are not considered to be bioequivalent.

Many pharmaceutical dosage forms have been designed to change the absorption profile of a drug by modifying its release. Such formulations are described in a number of ways: modified, sustained, targeted, phased, extended release, and prolonged action. All of them affect the rate and/or time at which drug is made available for absorption and will thus change the shape of the time vs. serum level curve compared with that produced by a conventional dosage form; however, after absorption has taken place, the original drug molecule will have identical pharmacokinetics to that in an unmodified release product. If the rate of drug delivery is a critical step in assuring efficacy or avoiding toxicity, modified release formulations should be used with care in previously stabilized patients and brand switches should be made with caution. The British National Formulary (BNF) currently advises that some modified release preparations containing diltiazem, theophylline, nifedipine, and lithium products may not produce the same clinical effect; where possible, patients should be stabilized on one brand.

One final factor determining the bioavailability of a given dose of drug is its chemical form. To increase solubility, stability, and sometimes both, many drugs are formulated as a salt, e.g., sodium with phenytoin or ethylenediamine with theophylline in the case of aminophylline. Thus a dose of 100 mg of each actually contains only 92 and 85% of the active compound, respectively. This is often referred to as the salt factor (S) and must be taken into account when calculating the actual dose of active drug received by the patient.

Drug Distribution

Following absorption, drug must find its way to the site of action. To be useful, this process must be much faster than the rate of elimination, allowing the drug to accumulate and exert its therapeutic effect. Distribution is determined mainly by the rate of blood flow to, and penetration into, the membranes and tissues of the target organ(s). As with absorption, the more lipid soluble the drug, the sooner it reaches the target. This is especially true of the BBB where the more lipophilic diazepam produces faster cerebral depression than lorazepam, but lorazepam has a longer duration of action because it remains at the site of action for longer, being less able to repeat the return transmembrane journey.

Most drugs reach their targets through extracellular fluid. Drugs must pass through capillary walls and into interstitial fluid to be able to interact with cell surface receptors, but this is an oversimplification when considering the behavior of individual drugs. In many cases, drug is concentrated through lipid diffusion (partitioning), ion

entrapment, or active transport mechanisms in various tissues, where action is thus prolonged.

How well a drug is distributed depends on a number of factors: the physicochemical properties of the drug (partition coefficient, potential for ionization, molecular size) and the characteristics of the target "compartment" (pH, fat content, volume, and vascularity). Once distributed, these compartments (e.g., fat, bone, muscle) may act as drug reservoirs, storing considerable quantities of drug. Up to 70% of a dose of thiopental deposits in fat within 3 h of dosing. Tetracyclines and biphosphonates can accumulate in bone. But accumulation in these compartments is not always adequately reflected in residual serum concentrations because concomitant metabolism and clearance have occurred. Such compounds do not lend themselves to therapeutic drug monitoring (TDM).

Traditionally, drug distribution to these various body tissues has been described by at least two imaginary compartments, largely distinguished by the extent of blood supply and the time the drug arrives there (see Figure. 2.2). The first compartment is considered to comprise of organs and tissues with a high blood supply, such as the heart, kidney, liver, lungs, and brain. The second compartment contains fat, muscle (mainly heart muscle in the case of digoxin), the peritoneal cavity, bone, and bladder. For many drugs, reaching 95% of complete distribution after a single dose takes about 2 h in bone and muscle (longer with respect to digoxin and heart muscle), 4 h in fat – which has a poor blood supply, but just 2 min in the kidneys. Drug is assumed to reach the second compartment by diffusion, with or without active passage, from the first. Where diffusion predominates, an equilibrium exists between drug diffusion to and fro between the first and second department. For certain drugs, it has been suggested that a third compartment, reached from the second, should be considered. This is only necessary when needing to describe the accumulation and subsequent removal of a drug in a sanctuary site or site of toxicity, for example, the inner ear with gentamicin.

Several factors can influence blood flow and sometimes redistribution between compartments. For example, exercise can increase cardiac output by some 5–6 times; patients on insulin may find a more rapid onset and greater extent of insulin action during a vigorous work out. Concomitant

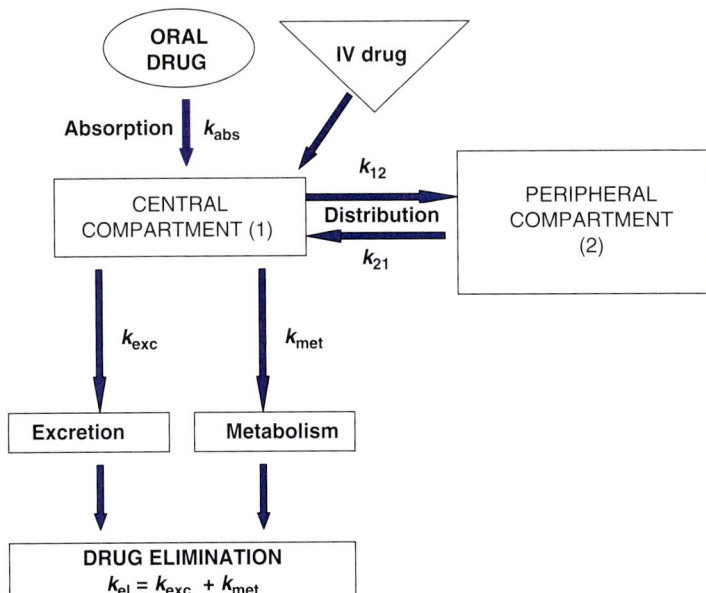

Drug movement can be described by a number of rate constants:

k_{abs} = the absorption rate constant; this can be manipulated by regulating the rate of delivery to absorption sites by, for example, administering the drug in a modified release dosage form or a depot injection.

k_{12} and k_{21} are the distribution rate constants between the first and second compartments At steady state equilibrium exists and they will be equal.

k_{el} is the elimination rate constant, comprised of the excretion rate constant k_{exc}, and the metabolism rate constant k_{met}.

disease can also have an effect; patients with heart failure are unable to perfuse tissues in either compartment optimally and drug distribution after absorption or from an IM injection site may be prolonged, thus delaying the onset of action and possibly the peak response for a given dose. Ischemia may mean that drugs acting on the target organ cannot reach it, e.g., the loss of efficacy of α-blockers in peripheral vascular disease. Poor renal perfusion may prolong the renal excretion of furosemide when used to treat heart failure, but as cardiac function and hence renal perfusion improve, lower doses may be required for further treatment.

Conditions such as shock can affect tissue perfusion and hence drug distribution; a decrease in drug clearance can also occur, due to reductions in renal or hepatic perfusion.

The division into two compartments is useful when attempting to explain the behavior of a drug

like digoxin, where the effects seen are related to serum concentrations, but only after equilibrium has been achieved between the first compartment, which includes blood and the second compartment, containing cardiac tissue. Digoxin is a relatively large molecule and it takes time (up to 10 h) for the equilibrium to be achieved. While the serum level target range of 0.8–2 μg/L (1.04–2.6 nmol/L) is usually taken as providing therapeutic levels in cardiac tissue, if the serum level is measured before distribution is complete, it will be too high compared to tissue levels and an overestimation of expected efficacy will be made. This is why a recommended gap of 8–12 h should be allowed between dosing (by whatever route) and serum level measurement (Winter 2003). We thus talk about digoxin behaving as if it were distributing into two compartments.

Figure 2.3 illustrates the behavior of a drug, like digoxin, which follows the two-compartment

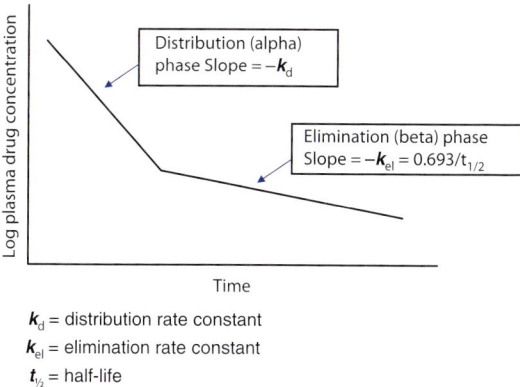

k_d = distribution rate constant
k_{el} = elimination rate constant
$t_{1/2}$ = half-life

FIGURE 2.3. Plot of log plasma level vs. time for a single oral dose of a drug displaying two-compartment pharmacokinetics, e.g., for digoxin.

model theory. After administration and subsequent absorption, which are relatively rapid processes, serum levels decline relatively rapidly due to distribution and elimination (called the α phase). This is then followed by a line with a shallower slope, representing the elimination phase only, termed the beta phase.

The practical implications of the two-compartment model are that any sampling for TDM purposes should be carried out after distribution is complete and that drug administration should proceed cautiously to avoid transient side effects due to high peak concentrations, which may reach equilibrium rapidly with target tissues in the first compartment.

For drugs where distribution is limited to the first compartment only, this is very rapid and there is no appreciable alpha phase. Other models with a third compartment have been proposed to explain the finer points of the kinetic behavior of some drugs; for example, a third compartment has been suggested for aminoglycosides where the patient has significant ascites or edema. The mathematics for quantifying drug behavior in such circumstances are complex! (Winter 2003). For most circumstances, one or two compartments will suffice.

Volume of Distribution (V_d)

We can describe a drug as being poorly or well distributed in the body, but it is sometimes useful to put a figure on this. First, to compare drugs with similar in vitro pharmacological properties, but

where differences in distribution might explain their differing potencies in vivo; and second, to help interpret differences in drug behavior within and between individuals that come about because of pathophysiological changes such as reduced plasma protein production, renal or hepatic disease, or heart failure.

In essence, the volume of distribution is a mathematical volume, relating the serum level of the drug to the administered dose in the following way:

V_d = Dose of drug (mg)/drug plasma concentration (mg/L)

Thus V_d is measured in liters.

A classic definition is that the V_d is the volume of fluid required to contain the total dose of a drug in the body at the same concentration as that present in plasma (Rang et al. 2003). V_d varies with body weight, and so for comparative purposes (and dose calculations when individualizing drug therapy!), literature values are frequently expressed as the specific V_d that has units of liters per kilogram.

For illustration purposes, Table 2.1 shows established, weight-related V_d values for a range of commonly used drugs. It also shows the extent to which the drug is bound to plasma proteins and the general lipid solubility or peripheral tissue binding affinity. Note that in general, drugs that are highly bound to plasma proteins with low lipid/specific tissue binding affinities have low V_ds; the reverse is generally true for drugs with high V_ds.

Note from the table that large, charged molecules such as insulin and heparin have low V_ds because they do not distribute well, being limited to a volume approximately equivalent to that of plasma. Heparin is a large molecule that is too large to cross the capillary wall easily and is thus confined to plasma.

Gentamicin and carboplatin are smaller, but still polar drugs that cannot enter lipid; these drugs also have low V_ds similar to the extracellular fluid volume (0.2 L/kg). Ethanol is a small, polar molecule and its V_d approximates to the volume of total body water (0.55 L/kg). More lipid-soluble drugs, such as morphine, propranolol, tricyclic antidepressants, and haloperidol, have greater lipid solubility and thus have V_ds that are greater than total body water. Digoxin is an interesting case in point. The molecule is relatively large and has polar centers, but has a V_d of 6 L/kg (an

Table 2.1. Examples of literature values for volume of distribution and plasma protein/tissue binding for a range of drugs used in critical care

Drug	V_d (L/kg)	% Plasma protein bound	Lipid solubility/peripheral tissue affinity[a]
Chloroquine	115	61	High
Amiodarone	66 ± 44 (SD)	97	High
Chlorpromazine	7	98	High
Digoxin	6	20	High
Amitryptyline	15	95	High
Propofol	4.2–14.3	98	High
Labetolol	3.4–10.7	50	Mod/high
Salbutamol	3.4	10	Unknown
Propranolol	2.3–5.5	80–95	Moderate
Metoprolol	3–6	12	Low
Fentanyl	3	84	High
Ciprofloxacin	2.5–3.1	30	Low
Quinidine	2.7	87	High
Clonazepam	2–4	47–82	High
Morphine	1.5–4	30	High
Lorazepam	1–2	90	High
Diazepam	0.5–2.5	97	High
Atenolol	0.5–1.5	<5	Low
Tubocurarine	0.3–0.6	40–50	Low
Midazolam	0.8–1.7	96	Moderate
Metronidazole	0.6–1.1	0–20	Medium
Teicoplanin	0.9	90	Unknown
Phenytoin	0.65	90–93	Medium
Theophylline	0.5	60	Low/medium
Carboplatin	0.25	24	Moderate
Valproic acid	0.1–0.4	80–94	High
Pancuronium	0.21–0.37	30	Low
Gentamicin	0.25	<10	Low
Meropenem	0.35	2–12	Low
Amoxicillin	0.3	18	Low
Vecuronium	0.3	90	Unknown
Imipenem	0.17	25	Unknown
Ceftriaxone	0.15	95	Unknown
Atracurium	0.16	82	Unknown
Warfarin	0.08–0.27	97–99.5	Low
Heparin	0.058	95	Low
Insulin	0.085	5	Low

Sources used: Dollery 1999; Rang et al. 2003; Anderson and Knoben 1997.

[a]Data comprises either of partition coefficient data or specific references to tissue binding capacity, where available.

Note that the highest specific V_d in the table for chloroquine represents an apparent V_d of approximately 8,000 L and the smallest, for heparin, 4 L.

apparent V_d of 420 L in a 70-kg adult), indicating extensive distribution from blood after administration. This is not because it enters lipid to any great extent, but rather it binds to muscle proteins, notable skeletal, and cardiac muscle, thus removing large quantities from the circulation. When you consider that the total volume of the adult body is only between 50 and 100 L, the impossibility of the apparent V_d representing an actual physiological volume becomes clear.

Amiodarone has one of the largest V_ds for any current therapeutic agent, although it is highly bound to plasma proteins. This is because the drug is very lipid soluble and also binds to a range of second compartment tissues, notably those rich in melanin. This reduces its concentration in body water considerably. The standard deviation for the amiodarone V_d, given in Table 2.1, illustrates the considerable interindividual variation that occurs due to variations in body lipid and melanin.

Use of V_d

Knowledge of V_d is useful in the following situations:

1. As a qualitative estimate of drug distribution as described above.
2. To calculate a loading dose; this is illustrated with the following example.

Calculate an IV phenytoin sodium loading dose to be given to a 72 kg patient to achieve a plasma phenytoin level of 15 mg/L (60 μmol/L).

The equation for the loading dose (LD) $= V_d \times C_p / S \times F$

S and F are the salt and bioavailability factors, respectively; C_p is the target plasma concentration.

$S = 0.92$ for phenytoin sodium; $F = 1$ (dose is given IV)

$$LD = \frac{(0.65 \times 72) \times 15}{0.92 \times 1} = 763 \, mg$$

The BNF states that the adult LD for phenytoin should be between 10 and 15 mg/kg (in our patient, 720–1,080 mg). Our calculated dose is therefore in line with standard advice.

3. To predict an initial plasma concentration after a given dose.

In the above example, if you knew the V_d and the dose, you could predict the plasma concentration after giving the loading dose.

4. To calculate the dose increase needed to boost a subtherapeutic level to a therapeutic one, the following relationship is used:

Required dose increase $=$ (target plasma conc.$-$ current plasma conc.) $\times V_d$

Caution when Using V_d

When individualizing drug therapy, one should always try and calculate V_d in the individual patient in question. This is easy if one has a recent steady-state blood level and a dose. As indicated in Table 2.1, literature values are widely available, but these are "average" or "normalized" values and can vary widely within an individual depending on the presence of comorbidities, age, gender, and body mass index. For example, the usual V_d for gentamicin, a water-soluble drug poorly bound to plasma proteins, is 0.25 L/kg. It may rise to as much as 0.3–0.4 L/kg in cardiac failure accompanied by ascites. It might also vary from day to day if the patient is in critical care suffering from fluid overload, depending on how this is managed.

A second thing to be wary of when using literature values is the format. In an attempt to "normalize" V_d, data are usually presented as the *specific* V_d with units of liters per kilogram. This has to be multiplied by the actual weight of the patient before using the resulting V_d to individualize therapy.

Drugs with poor lipid solubility are mainly confined to plasma and interstitial fluids; most do not enter the brain during acute dosing. Lipid-soluble drugs reach all compartments and may accumulate in fat. Drugs that accumulate outside the plasma compartment, either in fat or by binding to target tissues, may have apparent V_ds that greatly exceed total body volume; many of these will also have long elimination half-lives.

Caution should be exercised when trying to relate the V_d to the locus of pharmacological effect. As mentioned above, insulin has a V_d that suggests it distributes poorly away from plasma water, yet we know that it exerts its effects in the muscle, fat, and liver cells via receptors exposed to interstitial fluid but not plasma.

Drug Binding: Types of Intermolecular Bonds

Drug molecules usually consist of groups of atoms joined together with *covalent (electron sharing) bonds*. Such bonds are relatively strong, but they can be broken by hydrolysis, oxidation, or reduction. Such reactions require energy; they can be mediated through purely chemical means, such as the acid hydrolysis of peptide bonds, or the energy requirements can be lowered with the aid of an enzyme, for example, when the same peptide bonds are broken with the aid of peptidase enzymes. Similarly, drug molecules containing ester linkages can be degraded by hydrolysis, but also by nonspecific esterases in plasma, as is the case after administration of chloramphenicol succinate or atracurium besylate.

Ionic bonds, as the name suggests, involve the association of ions of opposite charge by the transfer of electrons from one to the other, creating an ion pair – one negative and one positive. Such bonds are weak compared to covalent bonds and are easily broken by the introduction of another ion of either charge, which has a greater affinity for the ion of opposite charge. Many drug molecules can form anions (or cations), loosing (or gaining) electrons in the process. Phenytoin is a weak acid, which at high pH, ionizes. It is then possible to form a salt (phenytoin sodium), which is a combination of negatively charged phenytoin and positively charged sodium. At high pH, phenytoin is water soluble, but if the pH is allowed to fall, for example by dilution with 5% dextrose for infusion, phenytoin free acid is formed; this is much less soluble and will readily precipitate. Ion exchange resins such as cholestryramine are capable of forming ionic bonds with bile acids and preventing their enterohepatic recirculation from the GI tract. Certain formulations of morphine contain the drug ionically bound to a cationic exchange resin; drug release is affected when morphine is displaced by ions in the GI tract.

In covalent bonded structures, electrons are seldom shared equally between the bonded atoms. One atom usually attracts electrons more than others, leading to a charge imbalance, or dipole. Such dipoles form weak, short-range attractions with other dipoles and ions. Such forces are called *van der Waal's forces*.

Hydrogen bonds are formed between very electronegative atoms, such as fluorine, oxygen, or nitrogen atoms and a hydrogen atom bonded to a similar sort of atom. Hydrogen bonds are stronger than van der Waal's and dipole – dipole bonds, but weaker than covalent bonds.

Van der Waal's bonds and hydrogen bonds play an important part in the way drugs interact with drug receptors, metabolic enzymes, and transport proteins, which in turn is determined by the molecular configuration in space. These forces also determine the degree of binding to plasma proteins, mainly serum albumin and α_1-acid glycoprotein, which can be a major determinant in the pharmacokinetic behavior of some drugs. Tissue binding is of a similar nature. Such interactions are reversible, concentration-dependent, and subject to competition from other binding species.

Plasma Protein Binding

One way that a drug may be held in the plasma compartment is by binding to plasma proteins; these are:

- Albumin
- α_1-acid glycoprotein
- Lipoproteins

Most weakly acidic drugs bind to albumin to a varying degree (see Table 2.1). Two binding sites are involved: site 1 binds drugs such as warfarin and phenylbutazone, and site 2, drugs such as diazepam and ibuprofen; drugs binding at the same site will displace each other in a competitive fashion. The binding is usually reversible, and at therapeutic concentrations, unlikely to be saturable, meaning that over normal therapeutic ranges, the percentage bound remains fairly constant. Three exceptions are salicylates, valproic acid, and tolbutamide. Here, addition of more drug will increase the free fraction disproportionately. Only unbound drug is free to leave the plasma compartment, diffuse across membranes, and enter target organs, including those where clearance takes place. Protein binding thus provides a reservoir of drug to replenish that removed from plasma in this way.

Protein binding can have a significant effect on pharmacokinetics. For example, unconsciousness occurs within 30 s following IV administration of thiopental and lasts for 20–30 min after a single dose. Rapid distribution to most vascular areas of the brain is followed by redistribution into other tissues and brain levels fall. Thiopental is strongly bound to plasma proteins, which impairs excretion through the kidney. The drug is metabolized to inactive compounds and then renally excreted. Thiopental, therefore, whilst having a short duration of action, may have a long elimination phase.

The extent of plasma protein binding is usually denoted as Fu, where:

Fu = unbound concentration/total drug concentration

This is often expressed as a percentage.

Protein binding also has its downsides, which are particularly important in cases where the drug is highly protein bound (Fu <5–10%). First, coadministration of a second drug that competes for plasma protein binding sites can reduce the bound proportion of the second drug leading to enhanced pharmacological effects. Endogenous compounds such as urea, bilirubin, and free fatty acids can also displace drugs from plasma protein binding sites and exacerbate matters. Drugs with high percentage protein binding shown in Table 2.1 are more likely to take part in clinically significant drug interactions.

Second, conditions that result in decreased synthesis of plasma proteins (e.g., liver disease, old age) or increased loss (e.g., nephrotic syndrome, severe burns) may result in hypoalbuminemia, resulting in increased free drug and pharmacological activity at normal therapeutic doses. In the critical care situation, sepsis can result in a rapid and profound decrease in serum albumin and subsequent redistribution of highly bound drugs.

Serum albumin is not the only protein involved. It is known that α_1-acid glycoprotein (acute phase reactive protein) binds drugs that are cationic at physiological pH, such as quinidine, alfentanyl, disopyramide, lidocaine, propranolol, imipramine, and erythromycin. It is known that stress of a critical illness, pregnancy, cancer, and inflammatory conditions such as rheumatoid arthritis, Crohn's disease, and hepatic cirrhosis can boost levels of α_1-acid glycoprotein and lead to increased binding of these drugs. For example, increased serum levels of quinidine have been observed following surgery or trauma (Fremstad 1976; Edwards 1982). Binding to α_1-acid glycoprotein can be saturated at therapeutic doses, e.g., with disopyramide. One might therefore expect to see exaggerated responses at high therapeutic doses or in overdose as a result; but many drugs are also bound to albumin and excess drug may be mopped up in this way. Although α_1-acid glycoprotein levels are seldom measured clinically, if elevated, serum levels are encountered, particularly with the drugs mentioned above and in the conditions listed, the possibility of raised α_1-acid glycoprotein levels should be borne in mind.

Significance of Protein Binding in Drug Interactions

Except in special circumstances, protein binding displacement does not result in increased drug effect. The age-old chestnut of warfarin illustrates the point that many putative drug interactions based on protein binding are of theoretical rather than practical importance. In theory, giving a second drug such as aspirin to a patient stabilized on warfarin might increase Fu from 1 to 2%. If that is all that happened, one might expect to see an exaggerated anticoagulant response. However, the body has ways of compensating for this. First, by increasing the rate at which the extra free warfarin is metabolized in the liver; on repeated dosing, this may take 3–5 half-lives to reach a new steady state. This assumes the absence of hepatic impairment. Second, the free drug is allowed to leave the vascular compartment in greater quantities and diffuse into other tissues, thus increasing the volume of distribution; this happens within a matter of hours.

In the above example, while there is an increase in Fu at the new steady state, the plasma concentration is decreased due to increased metabolism and V_d, but the unbound *concentration* remains much the same. What is more of concern is that at any concentration of warfarin, its anticoagulant action will be enhanced by the antiplatelet effects of aspirin; local bleeding due to gut irritation may also be enhanced. This interaction is pharmacodynamic rather than pharmacokinetic in nature.

There are two situations where clinically significant interactions involving displacement from plasma proteins have been reported. The first is where a high hepatic clearance drug (see below), such as lidocaine given IV for cardiac arrhythmias, is displaced. Almost all the drug is metabolized during the first pass through the liver. The higher the protein binding, the more drug is held in the plasma compartment, and therefore, available for metabolism. If a displacing drug is given, this increases Fu and the total plasma concentration falls due to increased distribution of liberated drug; in these circumstances, lidocaine clearance would fall.

Plasma protein binding is an important determinant of the rate of metabolism of phenytoin. In liver disease or nephrotic syndrome, where decreased albumin is accompanied by an increase in competing endogenous compounds such as bilirubin, Fu may increase from 0.1 to 0.35. A similar thing happens when competing drugs such as valproic acid are coadministered. In contrast to warfarin, there is often no compensatory increase in hepatic clearance because liver metabolic enzymes are saturated at therapeutic doses of phenytoin. Here, it is important for effective TDM to be able to assess the unbound phenytoin concentration, because it relates to therapeutic effect. It is usual to measure total phenytoin concentrations. Distinguishing between free and bound drug is expensive and currently carried out only in specialist centers. Limited advice is available on how to cope with such situations, for example, in end-stage renal disease and other cases of hypoalbuminemia (Winter 2003). When undertaking TDM of phenytoin in such situations, it is useful to envisage what the new therapeutic window would be, based on equations adjusted for the patient's measured serum albumin level expressed as a ratio to a normal population value.

In general, for any drug, the relationship between the plasma drug concentration and the plasma protein concentration can be expressed as follows:

$$\frac{C_{pat}}{C_{normal}} = (1 - Fu)(P_{pat} / P_{normal}) + Fu$$

Where: C_{pat} is the drug plasma concentration in the patient

C_{normal} is the normally expected drug plasma concentration with normal plasma protein binding

P_{pat} is the serum albumin concentration in the patient

P_{normal} is the normal albumin concentration

Rearranging the above, C_{normal} can be calculated for any drug

$$C_{normal} = \frac{C_{pat}}{[(1 - Fu)(P_{pat} / P_{normal}) + Fu]}$$

Hence, if the normal plasma albumin concentration is 44 g/L and Fu is 0.1 and the patient's total phenytoin plasma level is 8 mg/L (i.e., apparently subtherapeutic) and the patient's plasma albumin level is 25 g/L, substituting these values into the equation gives a normalized phenytoin level of:

$$8 / [(0.9)(25 / 44) + 0.1] = 13.1 \, mg / L$$

That is, the level is within the normal therapeutic range (10–20 mg/L or 40–80 μmole/L) and the dose need not be adjusted (although drug levels should be monitored closely).

Displacement by valproic acid is dose-dependent and also dependent on the steady-state phenytoin

level. When serum valproic acid levels reach 70 mg/L, sufficient additional phenytoin is displaced and thus available for clearance, to cause a fall in phenytoin plasma concentration of 40% (Winter 2003). Equations are available to calculate free phenytoin levels if one has levels for phenytoin and valproic acid in the same blood sample (Winter 2003). In such cases, it may not be possible to reach a definitive answer for an individual patient; however, the first step in solving any pharmacokinetic problem is to recognize that it exists and to work toward a sensible solution based on reasonable assumptions, using what credible information there is to hand – and with close monitoring.

Winter (2003) suggests some rules of thumb for helping to solve problems involving plasma protein binding:

- Any factor that alters plasma protein binding becomes clinically important when a drug is highly protein bound (Fu <10%).
- If Fu is >50%, then changes will have no clinical consequence.
- If Fu is increased in any given situation, the clinician should reduce the target concentration by the same proportion (Koch–Weser and Sellers 1976).

The blood-Brain Barrier

The BBB is a specialized layer of tightly packed capillary endothelial and glial cells with tight junctions between them, which act like a lipid barrier. Any drug targeted at brain tissue must pass through this; as it consists primarily of lipid, unionized, lipid-soluble drugs penetrate best.

The permeability of the BBB is, however, not uniform. The area between the general circulation and the chemoreceptor trigger zone is leaky, allowing the passage of some drugs that are excluded from other areas of the brain. This is helpful from a therapeutic point of view. For example, domperidone can cross the BBB here, blocking dopamine receptors to counteract nausea and vomiting caused by apomorphine when it is used to treat advanced Parkinson's disease. It cannot reach dopamine receptors in the basal ganglion where apomorphine exerts its therapeutic effect.

Inflammation can make the BBB more permeable, which is fortunate in the case of bacterial meningitis, allowing penicillin to reach the locus of infection after intravenous administration. Penicillin does not normally cross the BBB and would have to be administered intrathecally in the absence of inflammation. As inflammation subsides, so does penetration; hence, the first dose of penicillin is the most critical in this situation.

The role of PGP in drug transport across membranes has been described above; this helps to explain why some polar drugs seem to cross the BBB quite well, whereas some lipid-soluble drugs that are GP substrates are refused access. Some quinolone antibiotics, anticancer drugs, and loperamide show poor penetration, despite being highly lipophilic. Conversely, quinidine is known to inhibit PGP with the result that coadministration with loperamide produces centrally-mediated respiratory depression.

Drug Metabolism

Drug metabolism and renal excretion represent the two main pathways for clearing drug from the body. Drug metabolism takes place for the most part in the liver, but other sites may be involved, including the GI wall, lung, brain, kidney and in plasma (e.g., hydrolysis of suxamethonium by cholinesterase).

For most drugs, metabolism is a detoxification process, making lipid-soluble drugs more water soluble so that they are excreted in urine more readily.

For a few, metabolism converts an inactive precursor prodrug into the active, and therefore, more useful species (enalapril to enalaprilat). The sulfate metabolite of minoxidil is the active potassium channel activator responsible for lowering blood pressure in severe hypertension; azathioprine is metabolized to mercaptopurine.

For some drugs, the metabolite remains active for longer than the parent compound. For example, elimination of allopurinol is mainly by metabolic conversion to oxipurinol by xanthine oxidase and aldehyde oxidase, with less than 10% of the unchanged drug excreted in the urine. Allopurinol has a plasma half-life of about 1–2 h. Oxipurinol is a less potent inhibitor of xanthine oxidase than allopurinol, but its plasma half-life is far more prolonged (13–30 h); it is eliminated unchanged in the urine, but has a long elimination half-life because

it undergoes tubular reabsorption. Therefore, effective inhibition of xanthine oxidase is maintained over a 24-h period with a single daily dose of allopurinol.

Sometimes, the drug metabolites are more harmful than the parent compound, e.g., the oxidation product of paracetamol, N-acetyl-p-benzoquinoneimine is responsible for life-threatening hepatotoxicity seen in overdose. At therapeutic doses, the production of acrolein from cyclophosphamide results in hemorrhagic cystitis unless the antidote mesna is coadministered.

Metabolism can be divided into two phases (see Figure. 2.4). Phase one is catabolic in nature and involves oxidation, reduction, and hydrolysis. Phase two encompasses a number of synthetic (anabolic) reactions such as glucuronidation and sulfation where the metabolite is conjugated covalently with a more water-soluble compound. Many drugs undergo both processes; for example, a hydroxyl group introduced by hydrolysis in Phase 1 is a point of attack for a subsequent glucuronidation in Phase 2. Phenytoin undergoes extensive and complex metabolism; at least eight Phase 1 and two Phase 2 metabolites have been identified (Dollery 1999). Figure 2.4 illustrates the main Phase 1 and Phase 2 metabolic pathways for drugs.

To reach the microsomal enzymes in hepatocytes, drugs must be relatively lipid soluble to penetrate intracellularly. Water-soluble drugs are usually excreted without further modification because they are more readily excreted in urine anyway and cannot reach the microsomal enzymes in the first place.

Many drugs undergo Phase 1 metabolism followed by Phase 2, but this is not always the case. The route taken influences the potential for drug interactions. For example, midazolam is metabolized by CYP3A4, the major urinary and plasma metabolite being α-hydroxymidazolam. Midazolam will accumulate if coadministered with drugs that inhibit this enzyme. Lorazepam does not interact in this way because it is metabolized by direct glucuronide conjugation in Phase 2.

Hepatic metabolism can occur by non-P450 enzymes, e.g., via alcohol and aldehyde dehydrogenase, or xanthine oxidase.

Some drugs undergo metabolism at both hepatic and extrahepatic sites such as the lung, gut or plasma. For example, fentanyl is metabolized in the

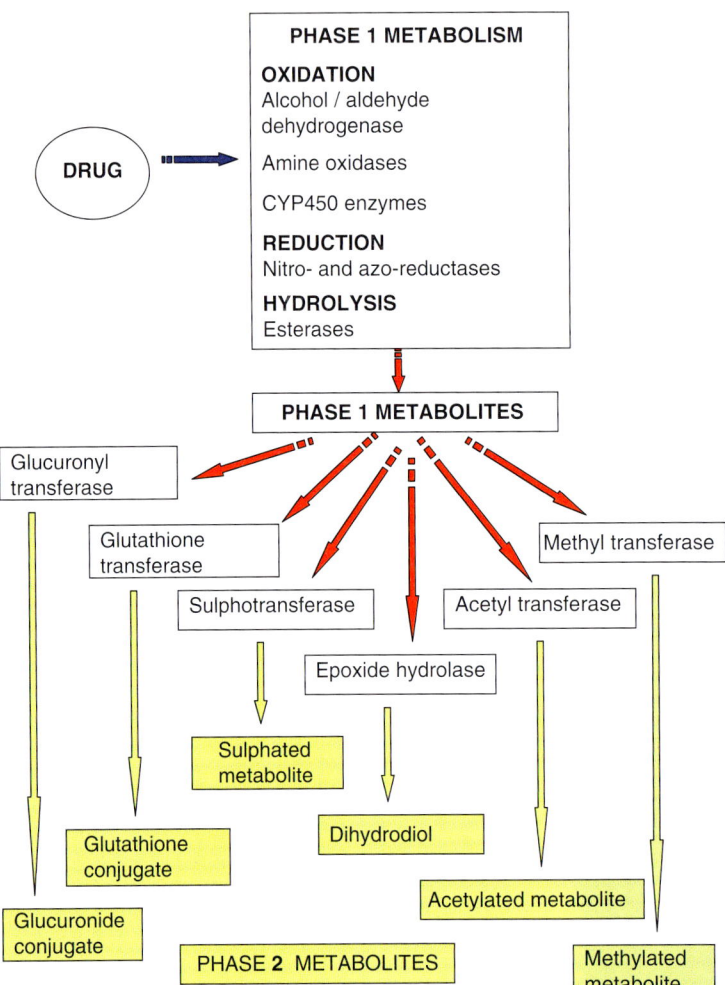

FIGURE 2.4. Main enzyme classes involved in Phase 1 and Phase 2 drug metabolism.

liver and in the intestinal mucosa to inactive nor-fentanyl by CYP3A4 isoforms. In this case, the potential of drugs to interact may be route-specific. If both drugs are administered orally, intestinal metabolism may be altered more than if they were coadministered intravenously.

Sometimes, metabolism is wholly independent of the liver. For example, the muscle relaxant atra-curium is administered as an ester, atracurium besylate. This compound is degraded spontane-ously by two pathways: a nonenzymatic decompo-sition process (Hofmann elimination) occurring at plasma pH and at body temperature and pro-ducing breakdown products that are inactive. Degradation also occurs by ester hydrolysis cata-lyzed by nonspecific blood esterases. Elimination of atracurium is not dependent on kidney or liver function and is useful in patients with renal or hepatic impairment.

The expression of certain hepatic metabolic enzymes is subject to genetic polymorphism. One clinically important manifestation of this is the emergence of two well-defined groups, one of which is comprised of individuals with low activ-ity of hepatic N-acetyl transferase and the other, normal levels of this enzyme. The so-called slow acetylators metabolize drugs such as hydralazine, procainamide, and isoniazid at a much slower rate than fast acetylators (e.g., the half-life of isoniazid is 100 h in slow acetylators and 40 h in fast acetyla-tors) with the result that these drugs may accumu-late in slow acetylators given normal therapeutic doses and predispose such individuals to a higher risk of drug interactions with drugs such as phenytoin and rifampicin (Romac and Albertson 1999).

Similarly, approximately 50% of a Western population is deficient in CYP2D6, meaning that drugs cleared by this mechanism may accumulate at normal doses, but that drug interactions involving this enzyme will not occur.

Stereoisomers

Sotalol, warfarin, cyclophosphamide, adrenaline, and bupivacaine are examples of drugs administered as racemic mixtures of optical isomers. Several clinically important drug interactions involve stereospecific inhibition of metabolism of one drug by another. In some cases, toxicity appears to be linked to one stereoisomer, which is not necessarily the pharmacologically active one. Where practical, regulatory authorities now urge that new drugs should consist of pure stereoisomers to avoid such complications. For example, cimetidine is a stereoselective inhibitor for the (R) isomer of warfarin, and when coadministered, should have a minor effect on prothrombin time, because the warfarin (S) isomer has the most anticoagulant effect. This is not to say that cimetidine does not enhance the action of warfarin – it is stereoselective but not stereospecific and some inhibition of the warfarin (S) isomer metabolism occurs. In contrast, metronidazole inhibits metabolism of the (S) isomer and significantly enhances anticoagulant activity. Other drugs that are stereoselective for the (S) isomer such as disulfiram and sulfinpyrazone or are nonstereoselective, e.g., amiodarone, will prolong the INR.

Phase 1 Metabolism

The cytochrome p450 (CYP450) family are responsible for most drug metabolism, and consequently, are the locus for most drug–drug and some drug–food interactions involving drug metabolism. The terminology derives from classification; for example, CYP3A4 gets its name from CYP (cytochrome), p450 (the most efficient nanometre wavelength of light used in assays, which incidentally results in pink coloration): 3 (family), A (subfamily), 4 (isoform).

Discovered over 50 years ago, CYP450 enzymes are a "super family" of heme proteins in a family of related but distinct enzymes, differing in their amino acid sequences. Each has a differing range of substrate (drug) specificities; CYP3A4 probably has the broadest. They each may be susceptible to a number of inhibiting or inducing agents and vary in their specificity for a particular substrate, although specificities may overlap. It is common to investigate the isoform specificity and potential for metabolism at an early stage in new drug development. Such information is useful in predicting not only the extent of metabolism, but also the effect of various diseases and coadministration of enzyme inducers and inhibitors, if their isoform specificities are known. The CYP system has been identified in the liver, GI tract, kidney, lung, and brain.

So far, 74 CYP families have been discovered, but most clinically important drug interactions in humans involve the first three – CYP1, CYP2, and CYP3. Ninety percent of therapeutic and recreational drugs are metabolized to some extent, by just five CYP450 forms in humans. These are CYP3A4 (40%) – the most abundant, CYP2D6 (20%), CYP2C9 (10%), CYP2C19 (10%) and CYP1A2 (10%). As a result, these five are major determinants of the intensity and time course of drug action and drug interactions and of variability of drug response between individuals. A further four account for most other drug metabolism: CYP2A6, CYP2B6, CYP2C8, and CYP2E1.

Table 2.2 shows a list of drugs metabolized by the CYP system and the main family members involved. The list is not exhaustive and the reader is referred to other sources for more complete lists. Exhaustive lists can also be found on the Internet (Flockhart, 2007) or in published reviews (Tredger and Stoll 2002).

Many drugs are metabolized by more than one enzyme, e.g., omeprazole is metabolized by both CYP2C19 and CYP3A4. Drug isomers can also be metabolized differently. For example, the (S) isomer of warfarin is metabolized by CYP2C9, but the (R) isomer is degraded by CYPs 1A2, 2C19, and 3A4. As the (S) isomer has the greatest anticoagulant activity, inhibitors of CYP2C9 will have the greatest likelihood of producing clinically significant effects (raised INR and potential bleeding). The reader should beware of attempting to apply in vitro, animal data to man. There are important differences in CYP regulation, expression, and composition between species. Also

TABLE 2.2. CYP450 drug specificities and interacting drugs

CYP450 enzyme	Substrate	Inducer	Inhibitor
1A2	Clozapine	Cigarette/cannabis smoke	Amiodarone
	Fluvoxamine	Oemprazole	Cimetidine
	Haloperidol		Ciprofloxacin
	Ondansetron		Clarithromycin
	Paracetamol		Fluvoxamine
	Theophylline		Ofloxacin
	Verapamil		
3A4	Azatidine	Efavirenz	Amiodarone
	Astemizole	Carbamazepine	Antiretrovirals
	Budesonide	Phenobarbital	Chloramphenical
	Chloroquine	Phenytoin	Cimetidine
	Ciclsporin	Neviparin	Ciprofloxacin
	Clozapine	St. John's wort	Clarithromycin
	Diazepam	Rifampicin	Erythromycin
	Fentanyl		Fluconazole
	Warfarin (R)		Fluvaoxamine
			Grapefruit juice
			Itraconazole
			Verapamil
2B6	Alfentanil	Carbamazepine	Orphenadrine
	Lidocaine	Phenobarbital	
	Midazoloam	Promethazine	
	Procainamide	Rifampicin	
2C9	Diclofenac	Quinidine	Amiodarone
	Glibenclamide	Rifampicin	Cranberry juice
	Ibuprofen		Fluconazole
	Losartan		Isoniazid
	Phenytoin		Lovastatin
	Piroxicam		Metronidazole
	Rosiglitazone		Sertraline
	Warfarin (S)		Zafirlukast
2C19	Amitriptyline	Rifampicin	Cimetidine
	Citalopram		Diazepam
	Omeprazole		Fluconazole
	Pantoprazole		Isoniazid
	Pantoprazole		Ticlopidine
	Rabeprazole		
2D6	Amitriptyline	Isoniazid	Antiretrovirals
	Carvedilol	Rifampicin	Fluoxetine
	Clozapine		Omeprazole
	Metoprolol		
	Risperidone		
	Thioridazine		
	Tramadol		
2E1	Paracetamol	Ethanol	Disulfiram
	Theophylline	Isoniazid	
	Ethanol		

Note: Some drugs are substrates for more than one CYP enzyme.

Clinically important drug interactions have not been observed for every possible combination in the Table; however, the information should provide grounds for caution when drugs from different columns are coadministered.

This list is not exhaustive; further lists can also be found on the internet (Indiana University 2005) or in published reviews (Tredger and Stoll 2002; Stockley 2002; individual summaries of product characteristics) beware of interpreting in vitro data to the in vivo situation. The rate and apparent specificity of CYP450 metabolism are concentration-dependent. For example, at high concentrations in vitro, amiodarone is metabolized exclusively by CYP3A4; however, at concentrations likely to be encountered by hepatocytes at therapeutic doses, both CYP3A4 and CYP2C8 are involved.

Not all Phase 1 metabolism involves the CYP group. Ethanol is metabolized by a soluble cytoplasmic, alcohol dehydrogenase enzyme and aminophylline and 6-mercaptopurine by xanthine oxidase. Monoamine oxidase inactivates noradrenaline and adrenaline.

Phase 1 reactions include oxidation and reduction. The CYP450 enzyme-mediated oxidation reaction requires sufficient enzyme, drug, and oxygen. The extent and rate of metabolism by this pathway may be reduced in patients with an oxygen deficit, for example, in chronic obstructive pulmonary disease, or where oxygenated blood supply to the liver is reduced, as is the case in congestive heart failure. Phase 1 metabolism of theophylline may well be reduced in these circumstances and maintenance doses may have to be reduced to avoid toxicity. Reduction reactions are less common, but warfarin metabolism involves conversion of a ketone group to a hydroxyl by CYP2D6.

Enzyme Induction

Table 2.2 lists some of the more important CYP enzyme inducing drugs. Over 200 drugs are known to cause enzyme induction. Many drugs are also substrates, and with time, accelerate their own metabolism (autoinduction) so that apparent tolerance can develop. This is important with carbamazepine, which is started at low doses and gradually increased to avoid toxic levels.

Many drugs are powerful enzyme inducers, e.g., ethanol, phenobarbital, carbamazepine, and rifampicin. Rifampicin can induce multiple isoforms (CYPs 2A6, 2C8, 2C9, 2C19 and 3A4); this drug also stimulates PGP, thereby decreasing drug absorption, which makes it a cause of clinically important drug interactions. For example, rifampicin causes loss of the immunosuppressant activity of ciclosporin by these processes.

Because enzyme induction requires gene transcription prior to the synthesis of additional CYP450 enzyme, interaction with a coadministered drug is not instantaneous. Onset of effect is likely to be seen within 24 h, but days may be required before the full effect emerges. What actually happens will depend on the dose of each drug, the time to reach steady state, and the isoenzyme affected. For example, the inducing effect of rifampicin is seen within a matter of days, but with phenobarbital, it can take a week or so. Most clinically important inducers are those given at high doses and/or with long half-lives. Similarly, when the inducing drug or other stimulus such as regular tobacco smoking is withdrawn, high CYP levels may take some time to resolve, so that increased metabolism of the first drug may persist for several days after discontinuation.

Enzyme induction has been exploited by administering phenobarbital to premature babies at risk of kernicterus. The drug stimulates Phase 2 glucuronyltransferase, encouraging the conjugation and thus detoxification of free bilirubin.

Some drugs are capable of inducing their own metabolism – a process called autoinduction. Carbamazepine displays increased clearance with chronic therapy, probably by induction of CYP1503A4, so clearance values derived from early dosing are of limited use when trying to predict a long-term dosage regimen. Furthermore, it is wise to initiate therapy at low doses and increase gradually, with careful monitoring.

Enzyme Inhibition

Table 2.2 lists some of the more important enzyme inhibitors. Inhibition of the metabolism of one drug by another usually results from competition for an existing quantity of metabolizing enzyme. Thus interactions can be fast in onset and manifest themselves within hours of coadministration of the interacting drugs and maximal at 4–5 half-lives of the coadministered drug. With exception of irreversible inhibition, resolution is rapid on withdrawal of the offending drug.

Inhibitors of CYP450 enzymes differ in their selectivity, reversibility, and in their abilities to act as substrates. For example, quinidine is a potent competitive inhibitor of CYP2D6, but is not a substrate for it. Fluconazole, itraconazole, ketoconazole, and miconazole are potent inhibitors of CYP3A4 that form complexes with the heme iron in this CYP enzyme. Fluconazole inhibits CYP2C9 at daily doses of 100 mg, but it takes doses of 400 mg to inhibit CYP3A4. Erythromycin inhibits both CYP1A2 and CYP3A4.

CYPs may also be inhibited by drug metabolites of, for example, clarithromycin, erythromycin, nortriptyline, lidocaine, and amiodarone. Effects may continue for several weeks after stopping amiodarone because of the long half-life. Some protease inhibitors are potent inhibitors of CYP450 enzyme subfamilies and HIV-positive patients, who are frequently taking multiple combinations of these drugs, are at increased risk of drug interactions.

One useful rule of thumb is that the higher the dose of inhibitor, the faster the onset and the greater the effect.

Drug–Food Interactions

Grapefruit juice can inhibit metabolism by down-regulating expression of CYP3A4 in the gut wall and liver. Drugs affected include terfenadine, ciclosporin, and several calcium channel blockers whose bioavailability is increased. Cigarette and cannabis smoke can induce CYP450 enzymes; so can Brussels sprouts. Most recently, flavenoids in cranberry juice have been shown to inhibit hepatic CYP2C9, allowing the accumulation of warfarin and subsequent clinically significant hemorrhage (Suvarna et al. 2003).

Metabolism at Nonhepatic Sites

There are appreciable quantities of CYP enzymes, notably CYP3A4, in enterocytes of the GI tract. These can form a formidable barrier to absorption and thus reduce bioavailability of drug substrates. This may partially explain why oral doses of ciclosporin are approximately three times higher than the required IV dose. Intestinal and hepatic metabolism of ciclosporin are approximately equal. This is an important site for clinically important drug interactions; for example, ketoconazole can inhibit the metabolism of ciclosporin here, leading to increased serum levels.

Phase 2 Metabolism

Conjugation reactions are possible if the substrate has a suitably labile group attached to it, such as a hydroxyl, thiol or amino group. Phase 2 is really a synthetic step that adds a large, polar moiety; however, the resultant metabolites are invariably inactive, less lipid soluble, and therefore, better able to pass into urine. The additional groups commonly encountered are the sulfate, methyl, acetyl, glutathione, and the sugar derivative, glucuronic acid. The glucuronyl transferase enzyme involved in this process has very broad substrate specificity and glucuronides of a wide range of drugs are produced in man. Most conjugation reactions occur in the liver, but the lung and kidney may also contribute.

Severe disease and poor nutrition impair Phase 1 metabolism, but Phase 2 is usually preserved.

First-Pass Metabolism

Mentioned also under bioavailability above, this term refers to the metabolism of drug received by the liver from the portal circulation. Drugs with high first-pass metabolism, e.g., lidocaine, metoprolol, propranolol, morphine, salbutamol, verapamil and nicardipine, are removed extensively from portal blood during their "first pass" through the liver after absorption from most of the GI tract. Such drugs are often referred to as "high extraction" drugs (see below). For such drugs, higher doses are required to ensure that sufficient drug reaches the general circulation to have the desired therapeutic effect. Marked interpatient variations in first-pass metabolism can mean that different patients need differing doses to obtain a similar effect. Hepatic disease can lead to an unwanted increase in systemic bioavailability; an alternative route of administration has to be chosen to ensure predictable dosing. Special dosage forms are required to deliver the drug to areas of the GI tract where the perfusing blood bypasses the liver and reaches the general circulation directly, such as the rectal or buccal/sublingual routes. Parenterally administered drug, including that administered by epidural and intrathecal routes, will avoid first-pass metabolism, as will drug administered percutaneously.

Drug Excretion (Elimination)

Drug excretion can take place via a number of routes. Anesthetic gases are eliminated by exhalation and some drugs and/or their metabolites undergo excretion into bile and elimination in the faeces. Small quantities of drugs may be excreted in sweat and saliva. The major route of elimination for most drugs is the kidney, either directly or as metabolites.

Relationship Between Excretion and Clearance

"Clearance" (Cl) is a specific pharmacokinetic term used to describe the rate at which drug is cleared, by whatever mechanism, from a particular volume of plasma. Clearance thus encompasses both renal and extrarenal (usually hepatic) clearance. Ultimately, drug will be eliminated from the body by whatever route, but it is extremely useful to be able to characterize the clearance mechanisms. Safe and effective dosing can then be based on this information.

For most drugs, clearance remains fairly constant. From a safety point of view, it may be better to use a drug that is cleared significantly by both renal and hepatic mechanisms (or neither), so that if the patient develops renal impairment, the liver can respond to clear more drug and prevent accumulation. Likewise, if the patient develops liver disease resulting in decreased drug metabolism, renal clearance mechanisms become more fully utilized so that serum levels of the drug do not rise. This is an oversimplification. It is known, for example, that the elimination of digoxin is mainly through the kidney as unchanged drug (60–80%), but some hepatic metabolism occurs (20–40%); however, in renal failure, doses of digoxin still have to be reduced to avoid accumulation and toxicity because, in general, hepatic metabolism of this highly polar molecule is inefficient. Clearance is essentially the rate constant in the following equation linking drug concentration (C) to elimination rate.

$$\text{Rate of elimination} = Cl \times C$$

Clearance (denoted Cl) is defined as that volume of plasma completely cleared of drug in a unit of time; it is usually expressed in liters per hour for drugs, but in milliliters per minute for the endogenous substance creatinine.

The total body clearance $(Cl_{tot}) = Cl_{metabolic} + Cl_{renal}$

And when the rate of drug administration equals the clearance rate, then "steady state" conditions are said to prevail.

$$\text{Rate of administration} = \text{rate of}$$
$$\text{elimination} = Cl_{tot} \times C_{ss}$$

Where C_{ss} is the steady-state concentration, which, if *first-order* kinetics prevail, will increase or decrease proportionately with alterations in dose regimen.

If treatment is stopped, then the blood concentration falls. The *fraction* of drug cleared in unit time is constant, with the result that the decay portion of the plasma drug level/time plot is curved. This is referred to as *first-order* decay and occurs with most drugs at therapeutic doses. For some drugs, notably at high dose where hepatic metabolic enzymes are saturated and hepatic metabolism is the major route of elimination, the *amount* of drug metabolized in unit time is constant and independent of dose. Here, the plasma drug level/time plot is linear (or *zero order*) and the line may have a very shallow, negative slope, leading to prolonged drug clearance, particularly in overdose. Phenytoin is an example where zero-order pharmacokinetics prevail in many patients taking therapeutic doses.

The elimination of drugs undergoing first-order elimination can be quantified in a number of ways.

Elimination rate constant (k_{el}) may be used. This is the fraction of drug eliminated per unit time. It is the ratio of clearance to V_d

Thus

$$\text{elimination rate} = k_{el} \times A$$

Where A is the amount of drug available for elimination.

Thus,

$$Cl \times C = k_{el} \times A$$

and

$$C = \frac{A}{V_d}$$

then

$$\frac{Cl \times A}{V_d} = k_{el} \times A$$

So

$$Cl = k_{el} \times V_d.$$

A plot of serum drug concentration vs. time would be curvilinear and be described by the equation:

$$C_t = C_0 \times e^{-k_{el} \cdot t} \qquad (1)$$

The term $e^{-k_{el} \cdot t}$ represents the fraction of the original drug concentration at time 0 (C_0) that would remain at time t after dosing. C_t is the remaining drug concentration.

Another useful concept for characterizing drug elimination is the half-life ($t_{1/2}$). This is defined as the time taken for the drug concentration to be reduced by a half. It takes approximately five half-lives for any drug concentration to decay to zero after stopping the drug. Similarly, it takes the same period of time for drug to accumulate to a steady-state concentration at regular dosing (repeat oral or steady infusion). Table 2.3 shows the influence of elimination half-life on time taken either to achieve C_{ss} or eliminate drug from the body; for most practical purposes, C_{ss} can be considered to be achieved after five half-lives have elapsed.

If we apply this concept to equation (1) above, then:

$$0.5 \times C_0 = C_0 \times e^{-k_{el} \cdot t_{1/2}}$$

and

$$0.5 = e^{-k_{el} \cdot t_{1/2}}$$
$$\ln(0.5) = -k_{el} \cdot t_{1/2}$$

$$-0.693 = -k_{el} \times t_{1/2}$$

Therefore

$$t_{1/2} = 0.693 / k_{el}$$

Note that $-k_{el}$ is the slope of the elimination phase of the plot shown in Figure 2.3.

Note also the reciprocal arrangement between $t_{1/2}$ and k_{el}; if you know one, you can calculate the other. Note also that $t_{1/2}$ will be patient-specific, because k_{el} is also patient-specific. We know that $t_{1/2}$ for gentamicin in an otherwise healthy adult with normal renal function is 2–4 h, but this may be prolonged to 24–36 h in a patient with severe renal impairment; so the dosing interval (but not the dose) is increased accordingly. Similarly, a patient with fluid overload may well have an increased V_d and half-life and require a greater dose, but administered less often to avoid accumulation. For most drugs, the aim is to achieve C_{ss} without wide swings in C; this is normally achieved by using dosing intervals that are similar to the normal elimination half-lives. Where this requires frequent dosing and patient compliance might be a problem, once daily, modified release formulations provide a means of slowing delivery, and hence, absorption

k_{el} and $t_{1/2}$ are thus useful for drugs displaying first-order pharmacokinetics. k_{el} can be calculated from the half-life and vice versa; or, if two plasma concentrations (C_1 and C_2) separated by time T are known, k_{el} may be calculated directly from the following equation:

$$k_{el} = \frac{(\ln C_1 - \ln C_2)}{T}$$

The half-life of a drug can also be estimated either by direct coordinate extrapolation from two plasma concentrations, one half the value of the other, in a curvilinear plot (not shown), or from the linear portion of a log plasma concentration/time plot shown in Figure 2.2, where the slope $= -k_{el}$.

Using the Concept of Clearance and Half-Life in Pharmacokinetic Equations

The following example illustrates how drug clearance can be used in pharmacokinetic calculations.

A patient needs digoxin to treat her atrial fibrillation. She weighs 68 kg and has a creatinine clearance of 49.2 mL/min. Calculate an intravenous loading dose followed by an oral maintenance dose.

A loading dose could be calculated as follows, aiming for a target digoxin plasma level of 1.5 µg/L:

$$Dose = \frac{V_d \times \text{plasma concentration}}{S \times F}$$

For IV digoxin, $S = 1, F = 1$

V_d = 3.8 (bodyweight) + 3.1 (creatinine clearance)

= 3.8 (68) + 3.1 (49.2) = 410.92 L

$$Dose = \frac{410.92 \times 1.5}{(1 \times 1)} = 616.38 \ \mu g.$$

Practically giving 600 μg.

To calculate the maintenance dose, we first need to calculate the digoxin clearance in this patient from the equation:

Cl_{dig} = 0.8 (bodyweight) + creatinine clearance

= 0.8 (68) + 49.2

= 103.6 ml / min = 6.22 L / hour

The change from milliliter per minute to liter per hour is essential; the target dose is expressed in microgram per liter and the half-life is in hours.

$$Oral \ maintenance \ dose = \frac{Cl_{dig} (plasma \ concentration)}{(S \times F)}$$

$$= \frac{6.22 \times 1.5 \times 24}{(1 \times 0.7)} = 320 \ \mu g / day$$

($F = 0.7$ for digoxin tablets)
Practically giving 312.5 μg/day

$$The \ half\text{-}life \ (t_{1/2}) = \ln2 \times \frac{V_d}{Cl_{dig}}$$

$$= \frac{\ln2 \ (410.92)}{6.22} = 45.79 \ h.$$

A drug accumulates on regular dosing. Table 2.3 shows the percentage of steady-state level achieved after successive half-lives. After five half-lives ($5 \times 45.79 = 229$ h or 9.5 days), 96.9% of final steady state will be achieved. To all intents and purposes,

TABLE 2.3. Clearance or accumulation of drug related to drug half-life assuming repeated dosing and the absence of a loading dose

Number of drug half-lives	Drug eliminated or steady state achieved (%)
1	50.0
2	75.0
3	87.5
4	93.8
5	96.9
6	98.4
7	99.2
8	99.6

this can be considered as steady state. In our patient, the loading dose rapidly achieves a therapeutic level of digoxin, which approximates to steady state; subsequent doses can be considered as fine tuning and maintaining therapeutic levels. Strictly, a steady-state serum level should only be taken after 9.5 days have elapsed.

This case illustrates some important points:

A target plasma level of 1.5 μg/L was chosen because this lies at the midpoint of the generally accepted therapeutic window of between 1 and 2 μg/L.

In the case of the IV loading dose, it may be prudent to administer this as two, 300 μg injections spaced 6 h apart, to allow the full effect of each dose to be assessed before more is given and help avoid toxicity triggered by high serum levels.

Equations used above for calculating digoxin clearance and V_d are taken from standard reference sources and derived from studies investigating digoxin pharmacokinetics in "populations" (sometimes quite small samples) of patients. They provide a reasonable estimate of what is actually likely to happen in this patient, but may be modified to account for comorbidity such as congestive heart failure (Winter 2003).

The final doses are determined after considering the results of the calculations in the light of what it is practical to give to the patient.

In the case of the oral maintenance dose, the best option is a combination of a 250 μg and a 62.5 μg tablet (total – 312.5 μg/day). It is an easy matter to back-calculate and determine what the actual plasma concentration should be.

Note the large volume of distribution calculated for this patient (over 400 L) – this is typical for this drug. Much smaller values indicate that a calculation or sampling error has been made.

In the first few hours after administration, digoxin serum levels bear no relationship to cardiac effect, so samples trying to establish this relationship should be taken at least 6 h after administration and preferably at the end of the dosing interval, just before the next dose.

In general terms, at steady state, we can determine the maintenance dose or steady-state plasma concentration as follows:

$$Rate \ of \ administration = \frac{S \times F \times dose}{T} = Cl \times average \ C_{ss}$$

Where T is the dosing interval.

From the above equation, it is clear that so long as S, F, T, and Cl are constant, proportionality exists between the dose and resultant steady-state concentration. Halving the oral dose or infusion rate should halve C_{ss}, doubling it will double C_{ss} and so on. Alternatively, to achieve a target C_{ss}, with constant S, F, T, and Cl, the above equation can be manipulated so that:

$$\text{new dose} = \text{new } C_{ss} \times Cl$$

Attention should be paid to units when calculating doses. If the target C_{ss} is in milligram per liter, then the new dose will be in mg; if C_{ss} is in micrograms per liter, then the calculated dose will be in micrograms.

The term C_{ss} in the above equations actually refers to "average steady state" C_{ss} and is adequate for most cases, but where knowledge of peak and trough drug levels is important in understanding efficacy and safety, as is the case with gentamicin, a more detailed analysis is required.

Assuming first-order kinetics, at steady state, the change in plasma concentration due to the administration of an IV dose will be equal to the change in concentration due to elimination over one dose interval:

$$C_{max} - C_{min} = \frac{S \times F \, \text{dose}}{V_d} \qquad (2)$$

Where C_{max} is the maximum serum level and C_{min} is the minimum serum level.

Substituting C_{ssmax} for C_{max} and C_{ssmin} for C_{min} in (1) gives:

$$C_{ssmin} = C_{ssmax} \times e^{-k_{el} \cdot T}$$

Where T is the dosing interval.
Substitution in (2) gives us:

$$\frac{S \times F \, \text{dose}}{V_d} = C_{ssmax} - C_{ssmax} \times e^{-k_{el} \cdot T}$$

So

$$C_{ssmax} = \frac{S \times F \times \text{dose}}{\left[V_d \left(1 - e^{-k_{el} T} \right) \right]}$$

$$C_{ssmin} = \frac{S \times F \times \text{dose}}{V_d \, (1 - e^{-k_{el} \cdot T}) \times e^{-k_{el} \cdot T}}$$

From the forgoing, it should be clear that k_{el} and $t_{1/2}$ will be useful when:

1. Calculating the time to steady state when giving regular doses, and therefore, helping to decide on whether a loading dose is required.
2. Estimating time to zero plasma level after stopping a drug, particularly when an overdose has been taken.
3. Estimating when to sample to obtain a steady-state drug concentration.
4. Estimating clearance/accumulation of a drug, and therefore, designing an appropriate oral or intravenous infusion regimen.
5. If the predominant organ of clearance is known, predicting the effect of organ disease on drug accumulation and elimination.

In all of the forgoing, first-order pharmacokinetic behavior should prevail.

Nonlinear Pharmacokinetics

Zero-order kinetic behavior is mentioned above. In this situation, clearance is capacity limited, usually due to saturation of hepatic metabolic enzymes. The most important drug here is phenytoin, where saturation often occurs at therapeutic doses. The reader might like to view alcohol in a similar light at this point. Particularly at the top end of the "dose," a quantity of drug, rather than a proportion of dose, is cleared in unit time, leading to accumulation and increased side effects. The pharmacokinetics of phenytoin require special mathematical modeling derived from the study of Michaelis–Menton enzyme kinetics and the reader is referred to specialist texts on this subject (Winter 2003).

A few drugs show increased clearance with increased serum concentration. This happens with valproic acid and disopyramide. In such cases, plasma protein binding sites are saturated at the top end of the therapeutic dose range, with the effect that a greater proportion of drug is metabolized, depending on the extent of increase in the unbound concentration.

Clearance by Specific Organs

Renal Clearance

To be able to quantify kinetic parameters in renal impairment, it is essential to have an appreciation of how drugs are cleared by the kidney and how renal function can be monitored. It is then possible to predict which drugs are likely to be affected by altered function (e.g., in kidney disease or disease resulting in reduced renal perfusion such as heart failure) and to make dose adjustments accordingly. A rule of thumb is that renal impairment will affect most of those drugs that are cleared extensively by the kidney when function is normal, such as digoxin, aminoglycosides, penicillins and cephalosporins, procainamide, amikacin, tobramycin, and lithium.

Some drugs (e.g., penicillin) are excreted rapidly and unchanged by the kidney after a single passage of blood. Other drugs excreted largely unchanged are furosemide, gentamicin, methotrexate, atenolol, and digoxin. Some, usually more lipid-soluble agents, are excreted only very slowly, e.g., diazepam.

Renal elimination has two mechanisms:

Glomerular Filtration (Passive Diffusion)

The upper molecular weight limit for drugs to be filtered into glomerular filtrate is about 20,000 (plasma albumin is about 68,000). Drugs highly bound to serum albumin, such as warfarin, are poorly excreted as a result.

Tubular Secretion (Active)

Two nonselective carrier systems operate in the proximal tubule. One transports acidic drugs such as methotrexate, thiazide diuretics, and furosemide, while the other handles basic drugs such as dopamine, amiodarone, narcotic analgesics, and amiloride. About 80% of drug delivered to the kidney reaches the distal tubule and it is a very efficient site for renal excretion of these drugs. As, unlike glomerular filtration, the carrier mechanism transports drug without an osmotic equivalent of water, more drug can dissociate from plasma proteins and make itself available for active transport. Secretion is rapid, and consequently, drug removal from blood is efficient, even if the drug is highly protein bound.

Some drugs can compete for the same transport system and inhibit each other's excretion by this mechanism (e.g., probenecid and penicillin).

Tubular Rediffusion

If a drug molecule is capable of passive diffusion, as is the case with lipid-soluble drugs, it can diffuse back from filtrate into blood by passive diffusion. In contrast, highly polar drugs can sustain concentrations in filtrate up to 100 times those in perfusing plasma; digoxin and aminoglycosides are good examples.

Many drugs are weak acids or bases and their degree of ionization will depend on urine pH. A basic drug will be more rapidly excreted if the urine is acidic, because once in the urine, more will be ionized and incapable of back-diffusion. Urine acidification has been used to encourage more rapid elimination of amphetamine. Acidic drugs will be more completely and rapidly excreted if the urine is made alkaline. This is the basis of administering sodium bicarbonate to alkalinize the urine in cases of aspirin and phenobarbital overdose and in cases of myoglobinemia, where an alkaline urine will increase solubility, and hence, clearance of this potentially nephrotoxic compound.

Measures of Renal Clearance

It is always extremely useful to know how well the kidney is functioning, particularly when this is a major route of elimination for the drug in question.

The term clearance is described above. Loss of glomerular function (either temporary or permanent) is the most important in limiting renal excretion of drugs. For some substances that are cleared by both mechanisms described above, clearance can be very high, e.g., for p-aminohippuric acid clearance is at the theoretical maximum for renal blood flow (700 mL/min). For others, clearance can be very small or nonexistent.

Creatinine clearance (Cl_{cr}) is a useful measure of renal function, because many drugs mirror clearance of this substance. Creatinine clearance remains relatively constant with unchanging health status, but is a sensitive indicator of deterioration in glomerular filtration. Serial serum creatinine measurements can assist not only in monitoring renal disease, but also in dosage calculation for drugs excreted by this route that require close therapeutic monitoring, such as digoxin and the aminoglycosides.

The measurement of Cl_{cr} from 24-h urinary excretion data is one of the most accurate methods for assessing renal function, but 24-h urine collection is time-consuming and may be inappropriate where renal function may be changing rapidly. Various formulae and nomograms based on body surface area, age, weight and gender have been advocated; for a detailed description of these, see Winter (2003). Creatinine can be measured in plasma relatively easily and the relation to renal function is well established and related to Cl_{cr} through the Cockcroft and Gault equations. When tested clinically, these equations have been shown to be one of the more reliable methods, at least in providing a first estimate.

"Male" equation:

$$Cl_{cr}(mL \,/\, min) = \frac{1.23\,(140-\text{age})\times \text{body weight (kg)}}{\text{serum creatinine}\,(\mu\,\text{mole}\,/\,L)}$$

"Female" equation:

$$Cl_{cr}(mL \,/\, min) = \frac{1.05\,(140-\text{age})\times \text{body weight (kg)}}{\text{serum creatinine}\,(\mu\,\text{mole}\,/\,L)}$$

These equations can be made more accurate in patients markedly lighter or heavier than 70 kg (±15 kg) by multiplying the calculated Cl_{cr} by a correction factor taking into account the patient's body surface area.

The correction is:
(body weight in kilogram) $^{0.73}$/70

The corrected clearance would be the calculated clearance × the correction above.

There are several important considerations when using the Cockcroft and Gault equations in a critical care situation. First, their use is limited to when renal function is stable; where it is changing rapidly, one is getting a snapshot of renal function at the time the blood sample was taken to measure serum creatinine. Second, while it is true to say that an inverse relationship exists between serum creatinine and Cl_{cr}, the relationship is curvilinear. Estimates become increasingly inaccurate above serum creatinine concentrations of 400–500 μmol/L (below a Cl_{cr} of approximately

20 mL/min); similarly, it is difficult to gain an accurate assessment of the change in Cl_{cr} when serum creatinine values are below 200 μmol/L (Cl_{cr} of approximately 50 mL/min).

Creatinine production is dependent on muscle mass, and in patients who have muscle wasting, have a long-standing illness such as cancer, who are elderly, have fluid imbalance or differ significantly from the 70 kg body weight on which the equations are based, calculations using Cockcroft and Gault will overestimate Cl_{cr}.

For example, a serum creatinine of 120 μmol/L in a 70-year old, 55-kg woman may represent an actual Cl_{cr} of around 30 mL/min. This is because in relation to total body weight, the muscle mass, and hence, creatinine production falls, compared to younger adults. The otherwise normal creatinine serum level is the result of creatinine accumulation due to poor glomerular filtration.

Another major limitation to the use of serum creatinine as an estimate of renal function is the time taken for serum creatinine to reequilibrate after sudden changes in renal function. It behaves like a continuously infused drug, and sudden, drastic changes in half-life (e.g., from 4 to 20 h following an 80% reduction in glomerular function, e.g., in shock) will mean that 4–5 half-lives will have to elapse before a new steady state is achieved (see Table 2.3); in this case, 80–100 h. This should always be taken into consideration when assessing the patient's renal status for the purposes of dose adjustment, and where possible, serial serum creatinine measurements should be performed to see the trend.

It is possible to estimate Cl_{cr} while serum creatinine is reequilibrating by using rather more complicated calculations based on two nonsteady state serum creatinine measurements, either by the use of customized equations (Winter 2003) or nomograms (Hallynck 1981).

The above methods are not generalizable to children. Although alternative methods have not been so extensively studied in children, one formula that has been advocated, at least for providing an initial estimate in children over 1 year old, is the following (Traub and Johnson 1980):

Cl_{cr} (mL/min/1.73 m^2) = 42 × height (cm)/serum creatinine (μmole/L)

Creatinine clearance is already adjusted to body surface area, and to obtain the child's actual clearance, proportional readjustment for the patient's actual body surface area is required.

Others have developed methods based on height and serum creatinine (Schwartz et al. 1976).

All such calculations should be made with extreme caution in critically ill children, where renal impairment, rapid changes in renal function, and low muscle mass are common.

Biliary Excretion and Enterohepatic Excretion

Liver cells secrete some drugs and their metabolites into bile, which is then excreted into the upper intestine. The transport mechanisms are similar to those involved in excretion in the renal tubules and also involve P-glycoprotein. If the drug is sufficiently fat soluble, it will be reabsorbed from the intestine and could regain the general circulation in sufficient quantities to reproduce a clinical effect, before returning to the liver once more. This "enterohepatic" circulation provides a means of prolonging the half-life of such drugs, and hence, their activity beyond what would normally be expected. Several glucuronide metabolites move in this way and are converted to the parent compound by hydrolysis before being reabsorbed from the intestine; examples include morphine, ethinylestradiol, and rifampicin. Up to 20% of the dose may be involved.

Some drugs such as vecuronium are excreted unchanged in bile without enterohepatic circulation, and for some, this represents the main clearance pathway. Rifampicin is mainly cleared by excretion of metabolites into bile that are not reabsorbed.

Hepatic Clearance

Hepatobiliary disease can affect the rate of elimination of many drugs, but our ability to make dose adjustments on the basis of hepatic function is imperfect. None the less, knowledge of ways in which hepatic impairment can alter drug disposition is clinically useful. The influence of drug and physiological factors on hepatic clearance and the relationships between them are shown in Figure. 2.5.

The liver is the prime site for metabolism, and hence, clearance of many drugs. Hepatic clearance depends on the following: the inherent ability of hepatic enzymes to amend drug structure, which in turn depends on drug structure itself; the rate at which drug is supplied to the liver in blood; and the amount capable of diffusing from blood into hepatocytes, which in turn is influenced by the degree of plasma protein binding. There are important complicating factors, such as the extent and type of coexisting hepatic disease and the ability of the drug or concomitantly administered drugs or other ingested compounds to induce or inhibit metabolic enzymes and extrahepatic diseases that alter hepatic blood flow such as portosystemic shunting and congestive heart failure.

Hepatic clearance can thus alter during the course of therapy for a number of reasons and it is often difficult to predict the cumulative effect of several of the factors mentioned above working in tandem. Take, for example, the case of theophylline. The "population" value for clearance is often quoted as 0.04 L/kg/h (Winter 2003). It is recommended that to predict the true clearance in an individual patient, this value should be multiplied by 1.6 if the patient is, or recently has been, a smoker, to account for stimulation of theophylline metabolism by constituents of tobacco smoke; incidentally, this also goes for cannabis smokers. If the patient has congestive heart failure, the factor is around 0.5, to account for reduced blood, and hence, theophylline supply to hepatic metabolic sites. This is a rough estimate and will vary with the degree of heart failure and success of therapy to treat it. There are also factors for coadministered drugs such as cimetidine (0.6) and erythromycin (0.75) that are known to impair theophylline metabolism and phenytoin (1.6) and rifampicin (1.3), which can induce metabolism, and hence, accelerate clearance. Winter (2003) advises that where several conditions coexist, the original clearance value of 0.04 L/kg/h should be multiplied by the product of all the relevant factors to arrive at the best estimate of actual clearance, but that the greater the number of additional factors, the greater the uncertainty in the clearance calculated in this way. The clearance may be a useful starting point, but actual clearance should be estimated in the patient once it is possible to measure serum levels resulting from a known dosage regimen.

Attempts to characterize drugs on the basis of whether they are "high or low extraction" drugs are only partially successful in practice. High extraction compounds are avidly metabolized by

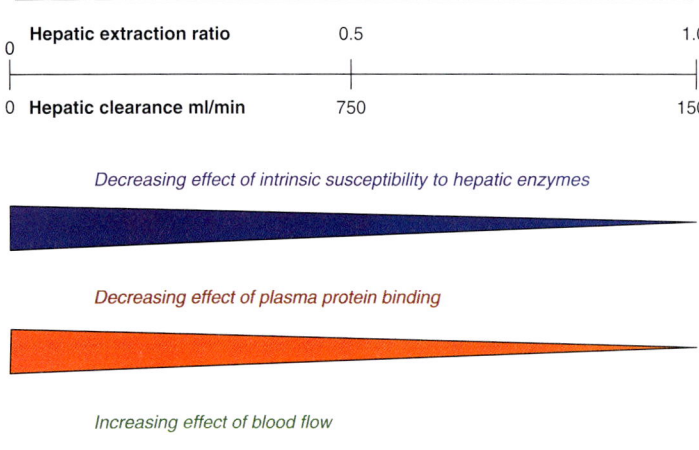

Low extraction	Intermediate extraction	High extraction
carbamazepine	desipramine	glyceryl trinitrate
diazepam	nortriptyline	lidocaine
phenytoin	quinidine	metoprolol
procainamide	paracetamol	morphine
theophylline		pentazocine
tolbutamide		propranolol
warfarin		verapamil

Hepatic extraction ratio 0.5 1.0

Hepatic clearance ml/min 750 1500

Decreasing effect of intrinsic susceptibility to hepatic enzymes

Decreasing effect of plasma protein binding

Increasing effect of blood flow

- For low extraction drugs, the clearance rate is lower than hepatic blood flow. They are often termed 'capacity limited'; the liver is extracting them as fast as it can, irrespective of hepatic blood flow.

- For high extraction drugs, the liver rapidly clears most of the drug presented to it, irrespective of the degree of protein binding; the only thing determining clearance is the rate of hepatic blood supply. These drugs are sometimes called 'flow limited'

Figure 2.5. Influence of drug and physiological factors on hepatic clearance (After Birkett 2002). The major determinants of hepatic clearance are blood flow, plasma protein binding, and intrinsic susceptibility to hepatic metabolic enzymes.

the liver, their clearance being largely determined by and sensitive to the rate at which they arrive there. The clearance rate of low extraction drugs is determined by the metabolic capacity of the liver and thus sensitive to diseases such as cirrhosis, affecting the mass of viable metabolic tissue. Drugs like theophylline are profoundly affected by a range of factors, e.g., reduced hepatic blood flow and reduced oxygenation of the liver, leading to reduced oxidative metabolism and reduced metabolic capacity. In many patients, these disorders coexist. This aspect is discussed further below.

Influence of Pharmacokinetics on the Choice of Dose Regimen

For most drugs, a one or two-compartment model is sufficient to describe their pharmacokinetic behavior (see above). This model comprises of a central compartment, taken to represent the blood and efficiently perfused organs, and a second compartment representing peripheral tissues and "depot" areas such as muscle and lipid. After absorption, drug passes into the first compartment and can only reach the second from there (see Figure 2.2). Drug must return from the second compartment to the first before elimination takes place.

A single dose of a drug with first-order kinetic behavior and displaying two-compartment pharmacokinetics will display the semilogarithmic plasma concentration/time curve shown above in Figure 2.3. Transfer of drug between central and peripheral compartments is often very rapid compared with elimination, so the slope of the first part of the curve, often called the α phase, is determined largely by distribution k_d. The slope of the line can be used to calculate a half-life of distribution. The second or beta phase of the curve represents elimination; k_{el}, and hence elimination half-life, can be calculated from its slope.

From the equations given above, it should be clear that plasma half-life is directly proportional to the volume of distribution and inversely proportional to the overall rate of clearance.

However, most drugs are not given as single doses, but on a continued basis to provide a target serum level. A continuous infusion can be regarded as the extreme of a repeated dose regimen; however, although all other regimens will be intermittent, the same kinetic parameters will be used to decide on the dose regimen required.

Taking the case of an infusion: after the infusion has started, the serum level will rise until the infusion rate equals the rate of elimination from the body – and the drug plasma concentration is steady. Regular, repeated intermittent injections or oral doses complicate the picture, but the principle is the same. The serum level will oscillate around an average steady state. Smaller and more frequent doses will alter the appearance of the plasma level/time curve toward that of a continuous infusion because there will be smaller swings in concentration. The exact dosage regimen does not affect the mean steady state or the rate at which it is approached. Steady state is usually reached within 4–5 half-lives. Faster attainment of therapeutic levels may be achieved by giving a larger loading dose to initiate treatment. This is particularly useful when the drug has a long half-life, but therapeutic control is required more rapidly than repeat administration of the maintenance dose can achieve; examples are digoxin, amiodarone, and phenytoin.

It should be remembered that phenytoin metabolism can become saturated at therapeutic doses, with the result that normal pharmacokinetic parameters cannot be used to describe its subsequent behavior. Steady-state plasma levels are no longer proportional to dose and elimination will be prolonged (see above).

Specific examples of dosage regimen design accompany sections on the individual drugs covered in this review.

Factors Affecting Pharmacokinetics

Physiological Factors

Most pharmacokinetic data provided in a successful marketing authorization application, and hence, the summary of product characteristics, are derived from studies on young, healthy male volunteers receiving doses of the drug covered by the license application, with the possible exception of elderly patients where data are now often required. By definition, critical care patients are not healthy, displaying a range of concomitant diseases that could mitigate against normal pharmacokinetic behavior; many are at the extremes of age and many receive doses outside the terms of the marketing authorization. The major physiological considerations are as follows:

Age

Drugs tend to produce greater and more prolonged effects at the extremes of age. The gastric pH is higher at birth (6–8) and may not fall to adult levels until the child is 2–3 years old. Thus the bioavailability of acid-labile drugs such as penicillin will be increased. For others, particularly weak acids such as phenytoin, it may be reduced. Other factors affecting absorption are reduced peristalsis and prolonged gastric emptying, leading to slower and less predictable absorption than in adults. Rectal absorption may be poor and erratic in children. The neonate has a greater proportion of body water than older children and adults, so the specific volume of distribution of water-soluble drugs such as the aminoglycosides is greater (0.35–0.78 L/kg in neonates compared to 0.2 L/kg in adults (de Hoog et al. 1998); thus relatively high doses are required to achieve therapeutic levels in neonates. Critical catabolic illness can result in muscle mass depletion and fluid overload, which can complicate the picture, increasing the adult V_d for gentamicin to 0.3–0.4 L/kg. The V_d of fat-soluble drugs would be lower in the neonate than in the adult. Muscle mass is low and blood throughput is poor, leading to reduced and unpredictable bioavailability from IM injection sites, especially in the presence of poor cardiac output. The larger ratio of body surface area to weight and more hydrated skin mean that transdermal penetration is enhanced, particularly for drugs with high intrinsic skin permeability such as corticosteroids; this can lead to adrenal suppression.

Drug binding to plasma proteins, including α_1-acid glycoprotein, may also be reduced in the neonate; in the elderly, drug binding to albumin may be low, but binding to α_1-acid glycoprotein may increase due to the presence of inflammatory disease or trauma that encourages its production. Highly protein-bound drugs such as phenytoin, furosemide, and indometacin will show an increased volume of distribution where plasma protein levels are low; conversely, where a drug binds primarily to α_1-acid glycoprotein, as is the case with erythromycin, a reduced volume of distribution would be expected. Fetal albumin has less affinity for drugs, resulting in high fractions of unbound compounds. Other conditions resulting from renal insufficiency, such as displacement from plasma protein binding sites by accumulating endogenous substances, metabolic acidosis, and hypoalbuminemia, are discussed below.

The BBB is functionally incomplete in neonates, allowing the passage of many drugs that are excluded in later life. Other factors altering permeability include acidosis, hypoxia, hypothermia, and inflammation of the meninges due to infection (Wade 1999).

In premature babies and neonates, renal function is relatively immature, slowing the clearance of water-soluble drugs such as gentamicin, lithium, and digoxin, and some drug metabolites. In the newborn, glomerular filtration rate (GFR) normalized to body surface area is only about 20% of the adult value. It increases markedly over the first 2 weeks of life, reaching similar values to adults at 6 months. Tubular secretion may take longer (8–12 months) to mature. For drugs that are mainly renally excreted, dosage adjustments involving magnitude and interval will be required. For example, flucloxacillin is recommended to be given at 12-hourly intervals up to 7 days old, then 8-hourly at 7–21 days, and 6-hourly thereafter (Royal College of Paediatrics and Child Health and the National Paediatric Pharmacists' Group 2003).

Renal impairment is a common presentation in the critically ill child, either due to coexisting disease (heart insufficiency), concurrent drugs (vasoconstricting inotropes), hypovolemia, and sepsis, or direct renal damage often caused by drugs. Assessment of renal function is often difficult, and in the critical care situation, made more so by rapidly changing renal status. Special care should be taken during this period. In some cases, empirical judgments, based on partial knowledge of pharmacokinetics in children and extrapolation from adults, are the best we can do. If hemofiltration or peritoneal dialysis is used, similar considerations to those used in adults with acute renal failure (see specific section below) should be made. In neonates, extended dosing intervals may be required because of this.

Renal function falls from early middle age onwards and may be substantially reduced (up to 50%) in elderly patients, despite apparently "normal" serum creatinine measurements. There is plenty of advice on dose modification on the basis of creatinine clearance in the BNF (Appendix 3) and individual summaries of product characteristics; but having made dose adjustments, the clinical situation should be carefully monitored for drugs with narrow therapeutic windows.

Drug metabolic capacity is still maturing at birth, so care is needed with drugs where hepatic clearance is known to be important such as diazepam, phenytoin, and theophylline. Both Phase 1 and Phase 2 metabolism are affected; neonates show immature metabolism by CYP450 enzymes, glucuronyl transferase, acetyl transferase, and plasma esterase, with "normal" adult levels being reached at about 8 weeks of age. The "grey baby" syndrome observed with chloramphenicol results from tissue accumulation of the drug due to slow conjugation in the liver. Similarly, morphine is not used in labor, because drug reaching the unborn child has a prolonged half-life due to slow conjugation, resulting in increased levels and prolonged respiratory depression. The development of kernicterus due to accumulation of free bilirubin has been associated with its displacement from plasma protein binding sites by competing drugs. The pathway for theophylline metabolism is different in neonates compared to older children and adults. In newborns, caffeine is produced rather than methyl uric acid. This can lead to caffeine toxicity unless lower doses are used. From about 1 year to the age of 9, theophylline clearance is faster than in adults due to the relatively large size of the liver; hence, larger doses per kilogram and shorter dosing intervals are used to ensure that therapeutic serum levels are sustained. The doses for aminophylline advised in the BNF illustrate this point: 6 months–9 years, 1 mg/kg/h; for 10–16 years, 800 µg/kg/h; and for adults, 500 µg/kg/h; adjusted according to plasma theophylline level.

In the elderly, reduced metabolism of many drugs could be a likely explanation for drug accumulation, although CYP450 enzyme activity declines slowly. This may be exacerbated by heart failure leading to reduced blood (and hence drug) and oxygen supply to the liver and a higher V_d for lipid-soluble drugs due to an increased contribution of fatty tissue to overall body mass. The increased half-lives of several benzodiazepines are evidence of these processes in action. Decline in these systems varies tremendously in the elderly population and if ever there was a case for individualizing therapy, this is it. It is more difficult to predict the level of hepatic function in the elderly, as metabolic capacity declines slowly and unpredictably with age; indeed, many elderly patients have the same capacity as younger adults. However, it is wise to anticipate reduced clearance of high extraction drugs such as diazepam and other benzodiazepines, and their active metabolites and to expect wide interpatient variation. The presence of concomitant disease, such as congestive cardiac failure, may strongly influence clearance, particularly for low extraction drugs.

Body Weight

Obesity and malnourishment can affect pharmacokinetic behavior markedly. If the patient is obese, the ratio of body fat to total body weight is increased, resulting in an increased V_d and half-life for lipid-soluble drugs and corresponding reductions in these parameters for water-soluble compounds. For water-soluble drugs, behavior is better correlated with ideal body weight (IBW). Calculations involving digoxin and gentamicin are based on IBW, rather than actual body weight in obese patients for this reason. It is appropriate to use actual body weight with lipid-soluble drugs.

Caution should also be exercised when assuming that a grossly obese patient has a degree of renal or hepatic function in proportion to their actual body weight; dose calculations based on an mg/kg basis should be made with caution.

Gender

With the exception of using variations of the Cockcroft and Gault equations to relate serum creatinine levels to clearance and minor variations in metabolic enzyme capacity, there are few important considerations to be made when comparing the pharmacokinetic handling of a drug between genders.

Pregnancy

Maternal plasma albumin is reduced and α_1-acid glycoprotein may be increased, influencing binding of drugs attracted to these macromolecules. Cardiac output may rise, leading to increased perfusion of the major clearance organs. As with any other biological barrier, lipid-soluble drugs cross the placenta with relative ease compared to water-soluble compounds. Drugs that do cross may accumulate in the fetus, either by binding to fetal tissues or because clearance mechanisms are far less mature than the mother's.

Genetic Polymorphism

There are clear examples of genetic variation influencing drug metabolism, and hence, drug response:

About 50% of the UK Caucasian population are fast acetylators of hydrazine-based drugs such as procainamide, isoniazid, and phenelzine and 50% are slow acetylators. The proportion of slow acetylators is lower in other races, e.g., the Japanese (13%) and Eskimos (5%). Slow acetylators are at increased risk of side effects if normal doses are used; they are more likely to suffer from peripheral neuropathy, which is due to isoniazid itself; whereas fast acetylators show greater hepatotoxicity due to the metabolite, acetyl-hydrazine.

Some individuals produce a variant of CYP2D6 that is inefficient at hydrolysis of debrisoquine, resulting in higher than expected levels at therapeutic doses.

Variations in plasma cholinesterase activity leading to reduced metabolism of suxamethonium have been noted. One in 3,000 individuals suffers, as a result, prolonged neuromuscular junction block.

Rare but important variations in phenytoin para-hydroxylase have been noted; this enzyme accounts for approximately 80% of hepatic metabolism of phenytoin and deficiencies could lead to accumulation.

Genetic variability in the ability to produce transporter proteins, e.g., PGP is discussed above. Low digoxin bioavailability has been linked with high levels of enteric PGP, which transports the drug back into the gut lumen through the intestinal wall.

The genomic profiling of individuals to determine single nucleotide polymorphisms that underlie these disorders is an area of intense research. This would allow us to assess their ability to metabolize a drug or better still, a battery of drugs, and in this way, determine which one would be best for them. A CYP450 "pharmacogenomic" test for variations in CYP2D6 and 2C19 is now available for in vitro testing in the EU and USA; but reports on its general applicability are limited (Clark 2005). In the meantime, we can at least recognize that variation in the ability to handle a number of drugs is determined genetically, and that as a result, the patient's response to a "normal" dose may not be as expected. In a limited number of cases, it may be possible to administer a "test" dose and measure the resultant serum level; but this might tell us more about the V_d of the drug rather than the rate or extent of metabolism.

Ethnicity

While many ethnic differences in drug response have been demonstrated, the majority are due to variation in pharmacodynamic rather than pharmacokinetic behavior. A clue that we know less than we should about this phenomenon comes from the observation that Chinese subjects metabolize ethanol differently from Caucasians, producing more acetaldehyde, and therefore, more flushing and palpitations. The example of differences in genetic polymorphism with respect to fast and slow metabolizers of hydrazine-like drugs has already been mentioned. This is an area where more research is needed; as such knowledge might be useful in predicting drug response along ethnic lines, or at least explaining it after the event.

Effects of Disease on Pharmacokinetics

Critical care frequently involves patients with multiorgan dysfunction, where the degree of dysfunction varies from day to day, hour to hour. An appreciation of the nature and extent of interference with the pharmacokinetic behavior is an important facet of care in this environment. Hemodynamic instability due to sepsis, shock, or dehydration can lead to multiorgan dysfunction and resultant changes in drug absorption, distribution, and clearance. Poorly adjusted mechanical ventilation can result in reduced cardiac output and blood flow to important metabolic sites such as the liver.

Renal Disease

Absorption

Acute renal failure may produce uremic neuropathy that reduces gut motility affecting the absorption of poorly soluble drugs and hyponatremia edema can lead to impaired drug absorption (Giles 1999a). In addition, poorly explained reductions in bioavailability have been reported for chlorpropamide, pindolol, and furosemide. Dehydration or salt wasting may affect diffusion to and absorption from, intramuscular sites.

Distribution

Acid/base disturbances may affect the ionization of weak acids and bases, their ability to partition into fat, and hence, their volumes of distribution. Acidosis can increase the concentration of unionized species of weak acids such as salicylate and phenobarbital, leading to greater CNS penetration.

Accumulation of nitrogenous waste products and free fatty acids, together with changes in acid/base balance, can displace drugs from plasma and tissue binding sites. Tissue binding disruption is a common cause of reduced V_d in uremia, as is the case with both loading and maintenance doses of digoxin. If normal doses are used, this can lead to raised concentrations in plasma with resultant risk of toxicity; dosage should be reduced.

In renal disease, serum albumin conformation characteristics change to the extent that affinity for some acidic compounds is reduced; decreased binding can be correlated with the severity of the disease. During sepsis, the integrity of the glomerulus is compromised and plasma proteins may be lost. These two factors can perturb normal pharmacokinetic behavior and are most likely to affect drugs that are highly bound to plasma proteins in the first place. For example, phenytoin can be as much as 30% unbound in uremic patients. Hydration status can affect the V_d for water-soluble drugs, e.g., gentamicin and meropenem.

Metabolism

The kidney is a significant site of metabolism for some drugs, such as insulin, morphine, salicylate, and digoxin; but the effect of renal disease on metabolism is poorly defined. Hepatic metabolic disturbances secondary to renal disease have been observed, e.g., reduced acetylation of isoniazid and procainamide; the cause is uncertain, but it may be related to uremia.

For certain drugs such as digoxin and perindopril, a decrease in renal clearance may be compensated for an increased hepatic metabolic clearance.

It is also worth remembering that drug metabolites may accumulate in renal disease. The importance depends on whether the metabolites are active, as is the case with propranolol and morphine or inactive, e.g., chloramphenicol. Fentanyl might be the opiate of choice in renal failure because its metabolites are inactive.

Drug clearance

With water-soluble drugs in particular, reduced clearance and increased elimination half-life can lead to some interesting problems, requiring a reduced dose and/or frequency for drugs with narrow therapeutic windows such as gentamicin and digoxin (Winter 2003). These aspects are discussed in more detail elsewhere in this review.

Dosage Modification in Renal Disease

This is a common clinical problem. Knowledge of the pharmacokinetics of the drug is essential and one should always look for experience of using the drug in renal impairment in the available literature or by consulting those with such experience (e.g., Bunn and Ashley 1999; BNF Appendix 3); but although the pharmacokinetic calculations are relatively straightforward, the clinical picture is complex.

The aim is to maintain the same average amount of drug in the body as would exist in a person with healthy kidneys. This can be achieved by reducing the dose, increasing the dosing interval, or a combination of these. For a bactericidal yet toxic agent like gentamicin, intermittent administration of normal doses is appropriate to achieve high peaks to ensure effectiveness and low troughs to prevent accumulation and toxicity. In the presence of severe renal failure, the calculated dose interval might become so prolonged (e.g., 36–48 h) that the serum (and hence target tissue) level is below the MIC for an unacceptably large proportion of the time. In such circumstances, a combination of reduced dose and lengthened dose interval might be the preferred approach. In the case of gentamicin, the drug must be given at intervals greater than its half-life in order to prevent accumulation and toxicity, so dosage adjustment can only be performed accurately by serum level monitoring and calculations based on first-order pharmacokinetics. Once-daily gentamicin dosing has gained wide popularity in recent years and is accompanied by special contraindications, monitoring, and interpretation criteria (Prins et al. 1993; Winter 2003).

For most drugs, serum assay is not readily available and dose adjustment must be done empirically; the following rules of thumb may help.

Most drugs tend to be given at dose intervals approximating to their half-life and this permits a simplified approach using the following equation:

Average amount of drug in the body

$$= \frac{1.44\,D \times t_{1/2}}{T} = \frac{D}{k_{el}T}$$

Where D = dose (mg), T = dose interval (hours), k_{el} = elimination rate constant (hour^{-1})

k_{el} is comprised of a renal component (k_r) and an extrarenal, metabolic component (k_m).

As total body clearance = renal clearance + metabolic clearance

$$k_{el} = k_r + k_m$$

(It is worth remembering that drug may be cleared by other mechanisms, such as excretion through the lung, through peritoneal dialysis, or hemofiltration; then the equation above would contain further elimination components, e.g., k_{lung}, $k_{dialysis}$, $k_{haemofiltration}$).

If F_{un} is the fraction of drug excreted unchanged in the urine, then:

$$k_{el} = F_{un}k_r + (1 - F_{un})k_m$$

The urinary elimination rate constant tends to be reduced in a manner proportional to the reduction in creatinine clearance (Cl_{cr}). So if we let the patient's Cl_{cr} represent a fraction (R_f) of normal renal function, the elimination rate constant under conditions of renal impairment (k_1) will be:

$$k_1 = \left(F_{un}k_r\right) \times R_f + (1 - F_{un})k_m$$

For the average amount of drug in the body under conditions of renal impairment to be the same as that under normal renal function, let

$$\frac{D}{k_{el}T} = \frac{D_1}{k_1 T_1}$$

Where D_1 and T_1 are the dose and dose interval in renal impairment respectively, then:

$$\frac{D}{k_{el}T} = \frac{D_1 / T_1}{\left[\left(F_{un}k_r\right) \times R_f + \left(1 - F_{un}\right)k_m\right]}$$

Therefore:

$$\frac{D}{T} = \frac{D_1 / T_1}{\left[F_{un} \times R_f + (1 - F_{un})\right]}$$

Rearranging;

$$\frac{D_1}{T_1} = \frac{D}{T}\left[F_{un} \times R_f + (1 - F_{un})\right]$$

Where $\left[F_{un} \times R_f + (1 - F_{un})\right]$ is the fractional dose adjustment, and degree of accumulation = 1/ fractional dose adjustment.

Consequently, the change in size of dose or length of dose interval is dependent on two variables: the extent to which the drug is excreted unchanged (F_{un}) and the residual fraction of normal renal function in the patient (R_f), expressed as $Cl_{cr}/120$.

The degree of accumulation can be calculated for various ranges of creatinine clearance and values of F_{un}. This is shown in Table 2.4. It can be seen that the degree of accumulation only exceeds 2 on certain occasions when creatinine clearance is *less than 50% normal* (60 mL/min) and Fu *exceeds 50%*. For many drugs, the fractional dose adjustment will be less than 0.5 only when these two conditions exist. For drugs with a wide therapeutic window, a dose adjustment larger than 0.5 will probably be unnecessary. Most pharmacokinetic adjustments for drug clearance are based on renal function rather than hepatic function because the latter is usually more difficult to quantify. For further information, see Giles (1999a).

Assumptions and precautions in adjusting doses in renal disease.

• The pharmacokinetics of the drug are first order over the intended therapeutic range.
• Metabolites are inactive and nontoxic. Patients with renal impairment who receive drugs on a medium to long-term basis run the risk of metabolite accumulation with subsequent toxicity. The consequences are difficult to predict unless previous experience is available.
• Apart from clearance, the pharmacokinetic profile of the drug (absorption, distribution, and metabolism) is unchanged by renal status. Plasma

TABLE 2.4. Degree of drug accumulation in renal impairment

% Excreted unchanged in urine (F_{un})	Creatinine clearance (mL/min)						
	0	10	20	40	60	80	120
10	1.1	1.1	1.1	1.1	1.1	1.0	1.0
20	1.3	1.2	1.2	1.1	1.1	1.1	1.0
30	1.4	1.3	1.3	1.2	1.2	1.1	1.0
40	1.7	1.6	1.5	1.4	1.3	1.1	1.0
50	2.0	1.8	1.7	1.5	1.3	1.2	1.0
60	2.5	2.2	2.0	1.7	1.4	1.3	1.0
70	3.3	2.8	2.3	1.9	1.5	1.3	1.0
80	5.0	3.7	3.0	2.1	1.7	1.4	1.0
90	10.0	5.7	4.0	2.5	1.8	1.4	1.0
100	∞	12.0	6.0	3.0	2.0	1.5	1.0

Degree of accumulation = 1/fractional dosage adjustment.
Fractional dosage adjustment = $[(1 - F_{un}) + (F_{un} \times R_f)]$.

protein binding is altered by uremia, notably for salicylates and phenytoin. V_d may be increased, e.g., for gentamicin, or reduced, e.g., for digoxin. Nonrenal clearance may be increased to compensate for reduced renal clearance; this is often seen as a safety net for drugs that are cleared significantly by both routes. In general, oxidative metabolism is enhanced, while N-acetylation may be impaired.

- There is no change in receptor sensitivity in uremic patients. Uremic patients may be more sensitive to the effects of phenothiazines, sedatives, and narcotic analgesics.

- Renal function is stable. In critical care and other areas where renal function may be changing rapidly, e.g., postsurgery, creatinine clearance should be assessed frequently and dose adjustments made accordingly. In a weakened, paralyzed patient, creatinine production tends to be decreased, and in catabolic patients, the reverse is true. In severe uremia, errors in estimating clearance may be large.

Renal Replacement Therapy

Factors to be considered when trying to predict the effect of renal replacement therapy on pharmacokinetics are shown in Table 2.5. Hemodialysis removes many water-soluble drugs and their metabolites quite efficiently, but because of its intermittent nature (e.g., 4 h, 3 times a week), the total amount of drug removed is relatively small. Normal drug doses are usually recommended assuming a GFR of less than 10 mL/min on dialysis and that timing of doses is independent of the dialysis schedule (Bunn and Smith 1990). If there is a perceived problem, doses may be given immediately after the previous dialysis session. The effect of critical care hemofiltration on drug clearance is less clear-cut and the topic of considerable research. Continuous hemofiltration may be associated with higher drug clearance; doses based on a GFR of 10–20 mL/min are frequently used. For further advice, consult specialist texts (Giles 1999b) or contact the manufacturers.

Liver Disease

Estimates of the degree of hepatic impairment, such as LFTs, raised bilirubin, and INR, should be available for most patients in critical care, but dosage modification based on them is imprecise. The best we can do is use them as signposts in conjunction with the known pharmacokinetic

TABLE 2.5. Factors to consider while predicting the dialysability/filterability and hence clearance of a drug during renal replacement therapy

Factor	Comment
Molecular weight	Drugs with molecular weights <30,000 Da will cross most high-permeability membranes. Drugs with molecular weights >500 will not cross conventional membranes readily
Aqueous solubility	Hemodialysis fluids will act as a sink for highly water-soluble drugs, which are cleared more rapidly
V_d	Drugs with low V_d are limited to the plasma compartment and are in contact with the dialysis membrane or hemofilter at high concentration. If V_d is >2 L/kg, clearance will be low; if V_d is <1 L/kg, clearance may be appreciable
Plasma protein binding	Low binding means high free drug levels ready to be dialyzed/filtered. Protein binding is commonly reduced in renal patients
Existing clearance	Drugs with high hepatic clearance (>500–700 mL/min) are unlikely to be appreciably affected by hemodialysis. In contrast, those where renal clearance is normally the major route, expect substantial dialysis. Dialysis mimics glomerular filtration, but not active tubular secretion. Expect greater removal if the usual mechanism is filtration, e.g., with fluconazole. Compensatory elimination by an alternative route may take place, e.g., hepatic elimination for ciprofloxacin
Half-life	Drugs with short half-lives (<1–2 h) will be removed more readily than drugs with longer half-lives. If one determines the half-life on dialysis using the equation $(0.693 \times V_d)/(Cl_{pat} + Cl_{dial})$ and this is less than the dialysis period, then the procedure will remove significant amounts of drug (Winter 2003)
Variations in dialysis equipment	Membrane/filter surface area, composition, porosity and susceptibility to clogging by cells and macromolecules in blood such as albumin can all affect drug and metabolite passage. Drug adsorption onto polyacrylamide filters has been observed with tobramycin, netilmicin, and amikacin
Dialysate	Composition, pH, molality, buffering capacity, and flow are all important factors
Technique	Blood flow, dialysate flow, duration, and intermittent nature will all influence drug removal

See also Anderson and Knoben 1997; Giles 1999b.

characteristics of the drug in question. For example, if it is clinically desirable to give a drug with a high hepatic clearance (extraction) value to a patient with cirrhosis, it should be started at a low dose, and drug levels and therapeutic/side effects should be monitored closely.

Drugs metabolized avidly by the liver are said to have a high extraction ratio (ER). Such drugs will experience marked reductions in metabolism if the blood supply to metabolic sites is reduced. Drugs with low ERs (<0.3) such as phenytoin, theophylline, and warfarin are less susceptible to reductions than drugs with higher ER values; their clearance is dependent on functioning enzyme capacity.

Alcoholic liver disease (cirrhosis) affects mainly flow-rate limited drugs as blood is shunted around the liver; dose reductions may be required for high ER drugs. For example, peak serum levels of labetalol and morphine may double in patients with cirrhosis. In severe hepatic cirrhosis there is reduced metabolic capacity, and portal-systemic shunting directs drug away from the site of metabolism. This can profoundly affect the systemic availability of some drugs such as chlormethiazole (×10) and pentazocine (×4). Reduced protein binding can lead to increased metabolism of the free drug fraction, and hence, increased hepatic clearance. Figure 2.5 lists drugs that have been characterized as high or low extraction drugs and illustrates the factors on which hepatic clearance depends. General advice on dose adjustment in hepatic disease is available in the BNF Appendix 2, the literature (Bass and Williams 1988) and some summaries of product characteristics.

Congestive Heart Failure (CHF)

CHF can affect pharmacokinetics in a number of ways. Drug absorption may be impaired due to reduced perfusion of the gut, resulting from a combination of reduced blood flow and mucosal edema. Reduced tissue perfusion will result in a reduced V_d for many drugs, e.g., severe CHF has been associated with up to a 50% reduction in the V_d for lidocaine. It follows that loading and maintenance doses may have to be reduced accordingly.

CHF will also affect renal perfusion, and hence, drug clearance by glomerular filtration; sluggish blood flow through the renal tubules may also encourage tubular reabsorption. Decreased hepatic perfusion may significantly reduce the metabolism of flow-limited drugs. Hypoxic conditions may affect the Phase 1 oxidative metabolic pathway. In extreme cases, negative inotropes have a similar effect on drug metabolism, e.g., propranolol can reduce the rate of lidocaine metabolism by this mechanism.

Thyroid Disease

Hyperthyroidism is associated with a general upregulation of metabolic activity, but the extent to which drug metabolism is affected is unpredictable. It is known that hyperthyroid patients are relatively resistant to the effects of digoxin and that hypothyroidism is associated with increased sensitivity. Digoxin clearance and V_d are roughly proportional to thyroid function, but the underlying mechanism is unclear.

Drug Interactions with a Pharmacokinetic Basis

Patients in critical care are at increased risk of developing drug interactions because of the multitude of medicines being used to treat multiple comorbidities with which they present; other contributory factors include the severity of disease, age, limitation on the choice of routes of administration, and multisystem organ failure (Romac and Albertson 1999).

Drug interactions having a pharmacokinetic basis are less easy to predict than those based on the pharmacology of the drugs involved – the so-called pharmacodynamic interactions. This is because pharmacokinetic behavior is determined by drug structure and by definition, each patented drug structure is different. Even within a class of drugs closely related in their pharmacodynamic effects, there are significant differences that determine parameters such as plasma protein binding, volume of distribution, and clearance. Any drug that is coadministered may cause drug-specific rather than general variations in any or all of these, with potentially important therapeutic implications; particularly where the drug has a narrow therapeutic window. Candidates can be found mainly among antithrombotic, antidysrhythmic, and antiepileptic drugs and lithium, and several antineoplastic and immunosuppressant drugs. Drug interactions are reviewed in detail elsewhere, but a few examples with particular reference to the usual suspects used in critical care will serve to illustrate that they can be classified in the same way as the topic of pharmacokinetics itself.

Drug Absorption

Absorption of orally administered quinolone antibiotics can be impaired by the coadministration of antacid preparations frequently administered to critical care patients. Warfarin and digoxin are bound by cholestyramine and bioavailability is reduced. Coadministration with enteral feeds can significantly impair the absorption of phenytoin and result in the failure of therapy (Bauer 1982; Parnetti and Lowenthal 1998).

Stimulation of CYP3A4 and PGP by rifampicin and St John's wort can lead to decreased absorption and/or increased metabolism of a range of substrates. Even though these agents may have been stopped on admission, their effect may endure for a few days to a week or so.

Drug Distribution

Displacement from plasma proteins is, under normal circumstances, not an important source of clinically important drug interactions. However, if the usual clearance routes are not available or plasma albumin is low, drug accumulation and toxicity may result. Caution should be exercised in coadministering drugs known to interact in this way to patients with significant renal or hepatic impairment. If the coadministration of both drugs is acceptable, the situation must be carefully monitored and it should be appreciated that the target concentration range of either drug may be altered as the ratio of bound to unbound drug determines pharmacological activity.

Special care is required if the displacing drug also impairs the clearance of the displaced drug, as is the case with salicylates, which not only displace methotrexate, but also compete for the renal anion secretory carrier. Quinidine, verapamil, and amiodarone can displace digoxin from tissue binding sites, while simultaneously reducing renal excretion and producing toxicity.

Drug Metabolism

This is the most important source of clinically important pharmacokinetic drug interactions. As mentioned above, clinical importance is difficult to predict in an individual because it relies on the pharmacokinetics of the two drugs concerned, their doses, the specific isoenzymes affected and whether those enzymes are being induced or inhibited. Table 2.2 gives examples of clinically important drug interactions; it is by no means complete. The reader is referred to specialist texts on the subject, the relevant summaries of product characteristics, and the references given in Table 2.2.

Drug Excretion

Drug interactions affecting renal clearance in the critical care setting are less well-documented. One classic is probenicid, which can block the excretion of a range of anionic drugs, including penicillins, by binding with the anion transporter protein responsible for their excretion in the renal tubule. Nephrotoxic drugs, like the aminoglycosides, can reduce GFR leading to accumulation of other drugs cleared renally, such as digoxin.

Competition between coadministered drugs for low-specificity transport molecules in the renal tubules can lead to clinically important drug interactions in the critical care setting. For example, coadministered quinidine can impair the excretion of digoxin, and together with impairing its metabolism, lead to a doubling of digoxin serum levels (Bigger and Leahey 1982).

Rules of Thumb when Dealing with Potentially Interacting Drugs

When dealing with patients who are receiving several drugs at the same time, it is important to observe the following rules of thumb to minimize the impact of pharmacokinetic drug interactions:

- Use drugs with well-characterized pharmacokinetic profiles.
- Minimize drug usage wherever possible and add new drugs only when absolutely necessary.
- Use all drugs at the minimum dose consistent with therapeutic effect and discontinue ineffective ones.

- Use drugs that can be monitored readily in plasma, preferably with wide therapeutic windows.
- Use drugs with an established relationship between serum level and therapeutic/side effects.
- Select a drug with the best practical knowledge and history of safe use.
- Use drugs with short half-lives to minimize the effects of drug-induced accumulation.
- Use drugs where there is evidence for two means of clearance, both renal and hepatic, so that if one route of elimination is impaired, the other may cope by clearing additional drug.
- If a drug interaction is observed, have a plan for dose adjustment to counter the effect of (a) continued coadministration and (b) readjustment of the maintenance dose of the first dose when the interacting drug is discontinued.
- Monitor the renal, hepatic, cardiac, and lung function closely, and recognize and respond promptly to changes that may exacerbate a drug interaction, such as reductions in renal clearance leading to accumulation.
- The time taken for a drug interaction to make itself known can range from minutes to months. In general, interactions resulting in a change in absorption, distribution, or renal elimination will occur earlier than those involving metabolism; in terms of drug metabolism, those involving enzyme inhibition will be recognized earlier (within a few days) than those involving enzyme induction (within a few weeks).

Deciding to Embark on Therapeutic Drug Monitoring

The following sections of this review deal with specific drugs for which TDM is important. A decision to undertake TDM is based on a positive response to any of the following questions. In critical care, there may be more positives than in other clinical areas.

- Does the drug have a narrow therapeutic window?
- Is there a variable relationship between dose and resultant serum concentration?
- Is there a good relationship between an easily-assayed fluid level (usually a blood level) and pharmacological response?

- Is toxicity suspected or anticipated?
- Are drug interactions suspected or anticipated?
- Is the drug being used where organ dysfunction is suspected or anticipated?
- Is the drug being used for prophylaxis (i.e., no clinical response to monitor but maintenance of a minimum serum level is necessary, as in the case of lithium or phenytoin)?
- Do product literature (SPC) and standard texts (BNF) advise the TDM approach?
- Does clear TDM advice exist for the drug(s) in question?
- Will TDM help with the pharmaceutical care of this particular patient at this particular time?
- Is TDM practical in this patient?

The last question is the cruncher. Being able to obtain an appropriate fluid sample for assay is just one of a host of factors that need to be considered if TDM is to be effective. Here is a check list of information required to optimize the effectiveness of TDM. In most cases, information will be incomplete; but using the principles discussed above, informed estimates can be made for some missing information:

- Accuracy and precision of the available drug assay.
- Expected time lag between sampling and result review.
- Time of last dose.
- Time of body fluid sample taken.
- Sample site.
- Dosage regimen and formulation used.
- Route of administration.
- Levels from previous samples, with all the detail from above.
- Units of measurement associated with the level (e.g., µg/mL, nmol/L)
- Patient age, weight or height, and gender.
- Pathophysiology and comorbidities, especially renal and hepatic disease.
- Pregnancy status.
- List of all other drugs taken, including dosage regimens, formulations, and routes.
- Other treatments, e.g., assisted respiration, renal replacement therapy.

Having decided to undertake TDM in the patient and advise on an appropriate therapeutic plan, subsequent drug levels should be monitored, correlated with clinical response and readjusted as required. It is worth remembering that many pharmacokinetic equations and published therapeutic windows are based on "population" data and should be considered as guidance only. For example, many patients remain seizure free on phenytoin levels of less than 10 mg/L and many will not suffer side effects above 20 mg/L, but will require the higher doses to protect against seizure. The maxim "treat the patient, not the level" remains sound advice.

Summary

This section has reviewed basic pharmacokinetic behavior and emphasized the importance of having as sound a knowledge as possible of the road map that drugs must follow to achieve the therapeutic objectives as efficiently and safely as possible. As with any map that is incomplete, informed guesswork based on the physicochemical properties of the drug, its formulation, coadministered drugs, and known patient morbidities can help.

References

Anderson PO, Knoben JE (1997) Handbook of clinical drug data, 8th edn. Appleton and Lange, Stamford.

Bass NM, Williams RL (1988) Guide to drug dosage in hepatic disease. Clin Pharmacokinet 15:396–420.

Bauer LA (1982) Interference of oral phenytoin absorption by continuous nasogastric feeding. Neurology 32:570–572.

Bigger JT, Leahey EB (1982) Quinidine and digoxin: an important interaction. Drugs 24:229.

Birkett DJ (2002) Pharmacokinetics made easy. McGraw-Hill Australia, Roseville.

Bunn R, Ashley C (eds) (1999) The renal drug handbook. Radcliffe Medical Press, Oxford.

Bunn RJ, Smith S (1990) Drug dosing during renal replacement therapies. Pharm J 244:413–414.

Clark C (2005) Patient profiling – the key to successful treatment? Hosp Pharm 12:446–447.

De Hoog M, Mouton JW, van den Anker JN (1998) The use of aminoglycosides in newborn infants. Paediatr Perinat Drug Ther 2:28–46.

Dollery C (ed) (1999) Therapeutic drugs, 2nd edn. Churchill Livingstone, London.

Edwards DJ (1982) Alpha-1-acid glycoprotein concentration and protein binding in trauma. Clin Pharmacol Ther 31:62.

Evans WE, McLeod HL (2003) Pharmacogenomics – drug disposition, drug targets and side effects. N Eng J Med 348:538.

Fremstad D (1976) Increased plasma protein binding of quinidine after surgery. A preliminary report. Eur J Clin Pharmacol 10:441.

Giles L (1999a) Acute renal failure. In: Elliott R (ed) Critical care therapeutics. London, Pharmaceutical Press, pp 31–48.

Giles L (1999b) Renal replacement therapy. In: Elliott R (ed) Critical care therapeutics. London, Pharmaceutical Press, pp 49–62.

Hallynck T (1981) Should clearance be normalised to body surface or to lean body mass? Br J Clin Pharmacol 11:523.

Hennessy M, Kelleher D, Spiers JP, Barry M, Kavanagh P, Back D, Mulcahy F, Feely J (2002) St Johns wort increases expression of P glycoprotein: implications for drug interactions. Br J Clin Pharmacol 53(1):75–82.

Hoffmeyer S, Burk O, von Richter O, Arnold HP, Brockmoller J, Johne A et al (2000) Functional polymorphisms of the human multi-drug resistance gene: multiple sequence variations and correlation of one allele with P-glycoprotein expression and activity in vivo. Proc Natl Acad Sci USA 97:3473–3478.

Flockhart DA (2007) Drug interactions: Cytochrome P450 drug interaction table. Indiana University, School of Medicine. http//medicine.iupui.edu/flockhart/table/htm. Accessed on 9 September 2005.

Izzo AA (2005) Herb-drug interactions: an overview of the clinical evidence. Fundam Clin Pharmacol 19(1):1–16.

Koch-Weser J, Sellers EM (1976) Binding of drugs to serum albumin. N Eng J Med 294:311.

Lin JH (2003) Drug-drug interactions mediated by inhibition and induction of P-glycoprotein. Adv Drug Deliv Rev 55(1):53–81.

Lown KS, Mayo RR, Leichtmen AB, Hsiao HL, Tugeon K, Schmiedlin-Ren P et al (1997) Role of intestinal P-glycoprotein (mdr1) in inter-patient variation in the oral bioavailability of cyclosporine. Clin Pharmacol Ther 62:248–260.

Malingre MM, Richel DJ, Beijinen JH (2001) Coadministration of cyclosporine A strongly enhances the oral bioavailability of docetaxel. J Clin Oncol 19:1160–1166.

Parnetti L, Lowenthal DT (1998) How to recognise and prevent dangerous food-drug interactions. J Crit Illn 13:126–133.

Phillips EJ, Rachalis AR, Ito S (2003) Digoxin toxicity and ritonavir: a drug interaction mediated through P-glycoprotein? AIDS 17(10):1577–1578.

Prins JM, Buller HR, Kuijpur EJ (1993) Once versus thrice daily gentamicin in patients with serious infections. Lancet 341:335–339.

Rang HP, Dale MM, Ritter JM, Moore PK (eds) (2003) Pharmacology 5th Edn. Churchill Livingstone, London.

Romac DR, Albertson TE (1999) Drug interactions in the intensive care unit. Clin Chest Med 20(2):385–399.

Royal College of Paediatrics and Child Health and the National Paediatric Pharmacists' Group (2003) Medicines for children. RCPCH Publications, London.

Shargel L, Wu-Pong S, Yu ABC (2005) Applied Biopharmaceutics and Pharmacokinetics, 5th edn. McGraw Hill, New York.

Schwartz GJ, Haycock GB, Edelman CM (1976) A simple estimate of glomerular filtration rate in children derived from body length and plasma creatinine. Pediatrics 58:359–363.

Stockley I (ed) (2002) Stockley's drug interactions, 6th edn. Pharmaceutical Press, London.

Suvarna R, Pirmohamed M, Henderson L (2003) Possible interaction between warfarin and cranberry juice. Br Med J 327(7429):1454.

Terwgot JMM, Malingre MM, Beijnen JH, ten Bokkel Huinink, Rosing H et al (1999) Co-adminstration of cyclosporine A enables oral therapy with paclitaxel. Clin Cancer Res 5:3379–3384.

Traub SL, Johnson CE (1980) Comparison of methods of estimating creatinine clearance in children. Am J Hosp Pharm 37:95.

Tredger M, Stoll S (2002) Cytochrome P450s – their impact on drug treatment. Hosp Pharm 9:167–173.

Wade P (1999) Neonatal intensive care. In: Elliott R (ed) Critical care Therapeutics. London, Pharmaceutical Press, pp 263–278.

Winter ME (ed) (2003) Basic clinical pharmacokinetics, 4th edn. Lippincott, Williams & Wilkins, London.

3
Introduction to Specialist Therapeutics

Kenwyn James, Spike Briggs, Rob Lewis, and Mike Celinski

- Drugs targeting the gastrointestinal tract in critical care
- Sedation on the intensive care unit
- Non-opioid analgesia within the intensive care unit
- Opiates in critical care.

Drugs Targeting the Gastrointestinal Tract in Critical Care

The gastrointestinal (GI) tract is a complex organ. Its significance in critical illness is being increasingly recognized and data from a large number of published human studies support the hypothesis that it contributes to morbidity and mortality in critically ill patients.

Gut dysfunction in critical illness can arise as a result of hypoperfusion or due to pharmacological and nonpharmacological interventions employed in the treatment of the illness.

The following conditions are associated with GI tract dysfunction in critical illness, and this article will review some of the pharmacological agents used in prevention and treatment.

1. Stress-Related Mucosal Damage
2. Gastrointestinal Motility Abnormalities (hypomotility, constipation, and diarrhoea)
3. Nosocomial Infection

Stress-Related Mucosal Damage

Endoscopically detectable mucosal erosions develop in 75–100% of patients within 24 hours of admission to the critical care unit. Overt GI bleeding has been reported in up to 25% of patients who receive no prophylaxis but clinically significant bleeding, defined as being associated with hemodynamic changes or requiring transfusion, occurs in only 1–4% of patients (Mutlu et al 2001). Mechanical ventilation for greater than 48 hours and coagulopathy are the major risk factors for clinically important bleeding and in the absence of either the risk is 0.1%.

Although stress-related mucosal damage (SRMD) is caused by the action of gastric acid, hypersecretion of acid is unusual in critically ill patients except those with head injury or burns. The prerequisite for acid in the pathogenesis of SRMD, however, makes gastric alkalinization the main goal in its prevention. Results on the relative efficacies of different drug groups vary greatly as do the opinions as to whether prophylaxis should be given to everyone or just those at high risk of significant bleeding.

Antacids

These are generally aluminium or magnesium-containing compounds that decrease gastric acidity by directly neutralizing the acid in a dose-dependent manner. In addition to their prophylactic properties, they have been shown to heal ulcers effectively in a manner independent of their effects on gastric pH. Suggested mechanisms for this include: binding of bile acids, inhibition of pepsin activity, promotion of angiogenesis in injured mucosa, increasing local prostaglandin synthesis, and the binding of growth factors, which increases their concentration at areas of mucosal injury.

M. Tomlin (ed.) *Competency-Based Critical Care*,
DOI: 10.1007/978-1-84996-146-2_3, © Springer-Verlag London Limited 2010

Magnesium-containing antacids cause diarrhoea. Aluminium-containing compounds inhibit intestinal absorption of phosphate and can cause significant hypophosphataemia. In addition, they can cause constipation and, particularly in those with renal impairment, aluminium overload which may lead to neurotoxicity and anaemia.

Sucralfate

Sucralfate is a complex polyaluminium hydroxide salt which has no effect on gastric pH, but provides a physical barrier to prevent mucosal damage by gastric acid. It does this by binding to the granulation tissue in exposed ulcer beds. This binding is greatest at pH < 3.5 due to the highly polar nature of sucralfate in acidic environments. It is thought that, in a manner similar to aluminium-containing antacids, sucralfate is also able to stimulate angiogenesis and localize growth factors to areas of mucosal damage. The combination of antacids and sucralfate should be avoided due to the potential formation of a solid mass or bezoar.

H$_2$ Blockers

H$_2$ blockers, such as ranitidine, increase gastric pH by blocking type 2 histamine receptors located on the gastric parietal cells and inhibiting acid secretion. Their effect on acid secretion, and therefore gastric pH, diminishes rapidly after 24 hours with a significant tolerance to IV ranitidine developing whether the drug is given continuously or as intermittent boluses.

The drugs are renally excreted and tubular secretion, in competition with creatinine, is important; mild rises in serum creatinine can occur as a result of this. The administered dose should be reduced in renal failure.

Concerns persist about the effects of increased pH on gastric colonization and subsequent nosocomial pneumonia. A large randomized controlled study comparing ranitidine with sucralfate, in patients requiring mechanical ventilation, revealed a trend towards a higher incidence of pneumonia in those taking ranitidine but this did not reach statistical significance. The same trial showed that those taking ranitidine had a significantly lower rate of clinically important GI bleeding than those taking sucralfate (Cook et al 1998).

Proton Pump Inhibitors (PPIs)

PPIs act by inhibiting H$^+$–K$^+$-ATPase enzyme in the gastric parietal cells. It is this enzyme that is responsible for the production of hydrochloric acid in the stomach. Proton pump inhibitors are activated by protonation in an acidic environment such as parietal cells when stimulated post prandially. This makes timing of administration important, and they should not be administered with H$_2$ blockers or other antisecretory drugs. This dependence on the activation of the enzyme for their effect explains why, unlike H$_2$ blockers, PPIs show increased acid suppression with repeated dosing, and decreased dose requirement to maintain pH > 4 with continued use. While pH value has not been shown to affect the outcome with regard to preventing SRMD, the ability of PPIs to produce and maintain pH > 6 improves clotting and may be beneficial in patients at risk of rebleeding from peptic ulceration.

The unprotonated drug is unstable in an acid environment and is usually given in an enteric-coated formulation; the high incidence of gastric hypomotility in critically ill patients therefore precludes the use of an oral preparation in this group of patients. Omeprazole (or Pantoprazole) can be given as an 8 mg/h dose for 72 hours or as a single daily intravenous dose of 20 mg for 3 days (Collier 2004). These regimes have been shown to reduce rebleeding in patients who have received endoscopic hemostatic therapy. They also reduce the number of units of transfused blood required, but no effect on mortality has been demonstrated.

The irreversible nature of their action requires new enzyme to be synthesized for acid production to resume. Following cessation of therapy, it takes 24–48 hours for maximal acid secretory capacity to return.

Gastrointestinal Hypomotility

Gastrointestinal hypomotility is common in critically ill patients, manifesting as delayed gastric emptying, decreased bowel sounds, ileus, or constipation.

Normal motility is dependent on the coordinated spread of waves of contraction and relaxation involving stomach and intestine, a process under the control of myogenic, neural (parasympathetic and sympathetic), and chemical factors. This migrating motor activity has been shown to be abnormal following surgery and in critically ill patients. Several factors including head injury, laparotomy, diabetes mellitus, hyperglycemia (even in nondiabetic patients), electrolyte abnormalities (e.g. hypokalemia), and drugs (particularly opioids, anticholinergic agents, and dopamine) contribute to this abnormal activity.

Delayed gastric emptying can result in intolerance of enteral feed, delayed absorption of drugs, gastric bacterial overgrowth, and gastro-esophageal reflux with the risk of pulmonary aspiration. This can lead to pneumonia and sepsis.

Metoclopramide

Metoclopramide acts on GI motility by antagonizing the inhibitory actions of dopamine at D_2 receptors. It also sensitizes the gut to acetylcholine and, therefore, vagal stimulation and increases the tone of the lower esophageal sphincter.

A 10 mg IV dose of metoclopramide, three times daily, has been shown to have a beneficial effect on gastric emptying when compared to placebo (Booth et al 2002). This effect on motility has not been demonstrated to have any beneficial effect on the incidence of pneumonia or mortality in critical care patients, although meta-analysis has suggested that 20 mg may be superior.

Metoclopramide has shown mixed results with regard to its ability to assist in the placement of postpyloric feeding tubes. A meta-analysis (Booth et al 2002) concluded that, on the available evidence, metoclopramide did not appear to provide any benefit under these circumstances.

Erythromycin

Erythromycin is a macrolide antibiotic that exerts its prokinetic effects by acting on motilin receptors in the GI tract. These receptors are found on parasympathetic cholinergic nerves as well as in the smooth muscle of the stomach and small intestine and, when stimulated, induce antral contractility.

Erythromycin has been shown to improve the chances of successful early enteral feeding and to significantly increase the successful passing of feeding tubes through the pylorus.

Other Prokinetic Drugs

Cisapride, a 5-HT$_4$ receptor agonist, has previously been used for its ability to increase gut motility. It is currently unavailable in the UK following its association with fatal cardiac dysrhythmias.

Opioids are extensively used in critical care. In addition to their desired actions, they are known to be potent inhibitors of GI motility, probably exerting this effect via peripheral mu receptors. *Naloxone* is a competitive antagonist at opioid receptors. When given enterally, naloxone selectively blocks peripheral receptors with minimal systemic effects due to its high first-pass metabolism. At a dose of 8 mg four times daily, it has been shown to decrease gastric tube reflux and the frequency of pneumonia in ventilated patients receiving opioid medication.

Neostigmine is an acetylcholinesterase inhibitor, and has been used to treat colonic hypomotility (Van der Spoel et al 2001). This supports the notion of autonomic imbalance with parasympathetic dysfunction in the development of these conditions. Neostigmine can cause bradycardia and bronchoconstriction, although low-dose continuous infusion appears to be associated with a lower incidence of this than higher dose bolus administration. Atropine should be available to treat unwanted effects.

Constipation

Reduced fluid intake, critical illness itself, reduced mobility, and drugs, such as analgesics, diuretics, calcium channel blockers, and anticonvulsants may all contribute to constipation in the critically ill patient.

Treatment includes the use of *senna, lactulose*, and *suppositories* or *enemas*. Senna increases intestinal motor activity as well as altering electrolyte transport across the intestinal mucosa. Lactulose is a synthetic disaccharide that exerts an osmotic effect due to the inability of the intestinal enzymes to metabolize it. However, certain colonic bacteria can split this molecule into two osmotic components that retain water and electrolytes in the bowel lumen.

Glycerine suppositories act by dissolving and softening faecal mass, so should be inserted directly into the faeces to have their effect. Generally, enemas also have a softening effect.

Diarrhoea

Diarrhoea is a common problem in critically ill patients. It has been reported to occur in up to half of all patients as a result of gut dysfunction from the critical illness itself, nosocomial infection, or as a complication of feeding or antibiotic use. The treatment depends on the underlying cause, but this is often complicated by an inability to identify this.

Probiotics are nonpathogenic microorganisms which, when ingested, exert a positive influence on the health or physiology of the host. These may work by stimulating the intestinal secretion of immunoglobulins, increasing brush border enzyme activity of intestinal cells, antagonizing the overgrowth of pathogenic microorganisms, and decreasing the intestinal secretion induced by some bacterial toxins. Probiotics may be beneficial in the treatment of antibiotic-associated diarrhoea, but may also have adverse effects in, for example, pancreatitis.

Nosocomial Infection

Critical illness is associated with marked changes in the patterns of microbial colonization. Such changes occur in the oropharynx and upper gastrointestinal tract due to a combination of reduced salivary flow, gastric alkalization, cholestasis, and gastrointestinal ileus as well as the use of broad-spectrum antibiotics. Pathological colonization occurs with the predominant nosocomial species, and descriptive studies have suggested that such colonization is a risk factor for infection. Viable microorganisms may trigger an infective process by the aspiration of the contaminated gastric or oropharyngeal secretions, or by direct passage cross the gastrointestinal mucosa, a process called bacterial translocation.

Selective Decontamination of the Digestive Tract

Selective decontamination of the digestive tract (SDD) is a treatment designed to prevent infection by eradicating and preventing the carriage of potentially pathogenic aerobic microorganisms from the oropharynx, stomach, and gut. The standard regimen consists of two components. Topical, non absorbable *Polymixin E (colistin), tobramycin,* and *amphotericin B* are administered as a paste to the oropharynx and as a suspension via a nasogastric tube. This combination is active against all aerobic gram-negative bacteria and fungi while having minimal activity against the indigenous anaerobic and gram-positive organisms which make up the normal gut flora. The presence of these organisms is thought to prevent overgrowth with the resistant bacteria providing the so-called colonization resistance. In addition, intravenous *cefotaxime* is usually administered for 4 days. The systemic treatment is to treat early established infection by community-acquired pathogens such as Streptococcus pneumoniae and Hemophilus influenza. SDD should be commenced as soon as possible following admission and continued until cessation of mechanical ventilation or discharge from the ICU.

Meta-analysis has shown SDD to significantly reduce the occurrence of ventilator-associated pneumonia and intensive care mortality, but it has not been widely adopted as a prophylactic measure in critical care units. One of the reasons for this is the continuing concern over the potential for the emergence of antimicrobial resistance. SDD does exert a selective pressure on MRSA and increased colonization with MRSA in SDD-treated patients has been reported (Schultz et al 2003).

Enteral Nutrition

Enteral nutrition has beneficial effects on the GI tract over and above nutrition. Early enteral nutrition started within 24–48 hours of admission to ICU improves nitrogen balance, wound healing, and host immune function. It also augments cellular antioxidant systems and decreases the hypermetabolic response to tissue injury. Direct GI effects of early enteral nutrition are the maintenance of mucosal immunity, prevention of increased mucosal permeability, and a decrease in bacterial translocation. Meta-analysis has confirmed this benefit to surgical patients in the form of a significantly lower incidence of infections and reduced duration of hospital stay. Enteral feeding appears to decrease the risk of overt GI bleeding, possibly by preventing SRMD via its beneficial effects on mucosal integrity.

Glutamine, in particular, is an essential nutrient for gastrointestinal epithelia. It has been shown to reduce or prevent gastrointestinal mucosal atrophy often seen during prolonged standard parenteral nutrition and is associated with decreased intestinal permeability. Despite this, animal models have shown mixed results with regard to glutamine's effect on bacterial translocation. Meta-analyses have suggested little benefit in infectious complications when enteral feed is supplemented with glutamine, with the possible exception of burns or trauma patients, but some benefit may be gained by parenteral supplementation at doses of greater than 0.2 g/kg/day (Heyland et al 2003).

Other nutrients, including *arginine, omega-3-fatty acids* and *nucleotides* have been shown to improve immune function in a variety of experimental models and have been used, along with glutamine, to enrich enteral feeding preparations producing "immunonutrition." These theoretical benefits are yet to translate to improved outcome with meta-analysis showing no effect on mortality, but mixed findings with regard to infectious complications and length of ICU stay (Heyland et al 2003).

Summary

Gastrointestinal tract function, as with other organ function, can be significantly disturbed during critical illness. Adequate oxygen delivery is not always immediately achievable which may exacerbate gastrointestinal dysfunction. This may result in SRMD and the possibility of haemorrhage, as well as gut hypomotility with its risks of delayed feeding and aspiration with resultant infection.

Pharmacological interventions are available for many of these problems although, as with many interventions in critical care, evidence is mixed regarding their effects on outcome.

Sedation on the Intensive Care Unit

Purpose

There are probably as many reasons for sedation as there are patients on the intensive care unit. Each patient is obviously unique and amongst many other needs, has their own personal requirements for sedation. Sedation should therefore be tailored to the individual's clinical and holistic situation.

There are broad purposes for sedating patients on the intensive care unit. The use and acceptability of these purposes varies between countries and individual intensive care units. However, reasonable sedation may be perceived to be a part of compassionate care of the patient by the clinical team. It helps the patient to cope with intolerable

conditions, coupled with stress and anxiety when faced with life-threatening circumstances.

The more frequent reasons for sedation are outlined below:

- Treatment of specific conditions such as
  - Epilepsy
  - Raised intracranial pressure
  - Tetanus
- Amnesia – obliteration of unpleasant memories of events such as injuries, procedures, and invasive treatment, and enforced passivity
- Reduction in unpleasant sensations – dry mouth, thirst, relatively static position, physiotherapy, tracheal intubation, tracheal suction, mechanical ventilation
- Allaying of anxiety – seen as a humane act to someone in keen distress
- Sleep – attempts to normalize sleep patterns are seen as beneficial, although difficult to achieve through the use of sedation
- Restraint and safety – physical restraints are acceptable in some countries and units, while chemical restraint is used in others. Restraint is sometimes necessary to protect the patient from self-inflicted injuries, and also to prevent injuries to the carers
- Reduction of stress – useful in reducing catecholamine output, reducing pulse rate and blood pressure, thereby reducing myocardial oxygen demand
- Reduction of metabolic demand – reducing carbon dioxide production and oxygen demand, and reducing nutritional demand
- Reduction and control of the symptoms of withdrawal from previously administered drugs

Objective

Sedation may be defined as a state of reduced consciousness where verbal contact with the patient is maintained. Plainly, on the intensive care unit, patients are frequently anesthetized, rather than just sedated, and are unresponsive to any stimulus. On occasion, such an anesthetized state is desirable, such as during tracheal intubation, insertion of tracheostomy, and control of intransigent raised intracranial pressure. However, oversedation used routinely on the intensive care unit is undesirable, and is associated with:

- An increase in nosocomial infections
- Cardiovascular depression
- More frequent neurological assessments including computed axial tomography scans
- A longer stay in intensive care unit and in hospital
- An increased incidence of postintensive care, psychological problems such as posttraumatic stress disorder and depression
- A greater cost of drug therapy

The objective of sedating a patient should be clear to the caring team, and may be protocolized to help minimize the negative effects outlined above, while achieving the desired outcome for the patient. This desired outcome should be a peaceful patient, who is cooperative, and responds to commands, and who occasionally requires deeper sedation for unpleasant procedures. Accomplishing these aims may involve not only drug-induced sedation, but also other strategies such as maintaining good, positive communication with the patient, frequent contact between patient and friends and relatives, relief of unpleasant circumstances, and avoidance of distressing situations.

Some sedatives, particularly those with long half-lives, may accumulate over a period of time. Accumulation will be more pronounced when these drugs are given by infusion, and when decreased renal and hepatic function reduce the rate of elimination of the drug and active metabolites.

Incorporation of a sedation-free period each day has been shown to reduce some of the negative aspects of sedation outlined above. Sedation is withdrawn for a period until the patient either "wakes-up," or attains a certain level of responsiveness.

The level of sedation may be assessed by a number of methods:

- The Ramsay score provides a subjective six point score of the depth of sedation. This is one of a number of sedation scoring systems. Certainly, one of the advantages of such systems is that sedation is looked at critically on a regular basis
- The electroencephalograph may be used to measure electrical brain activity, particularly when using barbiturates to control epilepsy. The data may be processed and presented in a number of forms, such as the bispectral index
- Evoked auditory potentials are used to monitor the depth of anesthesia

The Ideal Sedative Agent

There is no such thing as an ideal sedative agent. However, consideration of the attributes of such an agent is instructive when assessing the agents to hand on the intensive care unit, and selecting the appropriate one for a particular patient.

The attributes of an ideal sedative agent would include the following:

- Rapid onset and offset
- Induces sleep, amnesia, and anxiolysis in combination or singly
- No accumulation
- Cardiovascularly stable
- Avoids respiratory depression
- Nontoxic and zero incidence of anaphylaxis
- No inducement of tolerance
- Nonreliant on renal or hepatic function for elimination
- No long-term effects in terms of memory, dependence, psychological effects
- Easy to store at room temperature for long periods
- Economic

Considerable progress has been made towards this ideal during the past few decades, but all the agents in use today have some degree of unwanted and potentially harmful effect on the patient.

Sedative Agents

Benzodiazepines

This class of sedatives is one of the most widely used on the intensive care unit. They act through specific benzodiazepine receptors that are widely distributed through the central nervous system (CNS). These receptors are closely associated with GABA receptors, and are thought to work in a similar manner, whereby once activated, chloride ion channels open, resulting in hyperpolarized neuronal cell membranes, reducing synaptic transmission of impulses.

The main actions of benzodiazepines are:

- Sedation
- Anxiolysis
- Anterograde amnesia
- Anticonvulsant therapy

Benzodiazepines are metabolized in the liver, and in some cases, the metabolites are pharmacologically active, with particularly long elimination half-lives. A cumulative effect is quite likely in patients with renal and hepatic dysfunction, and therefore care is required when using these drugs, particularly by infusion.

Benzodiazepines are commonly used in combination with opioids, taking advantage of the synergistic effect. This enables the objectives of sedation to be achieved at lower dosage levels, reducing unwanted side effects.

These drugs may produce severe cardiopulmonary depression in the critically ill, and require careful experienced use in these patients.

• Midazolam

This is a short-acting benzodiazepine (elimination half-life of up to 3.5 h), administered by either bolus injection (up to 0.1 mg/kg for induction of anesthesia) or by infusion (0.02–0.2 mg/kg/h). There is quite a variation of dosage between patients, and thus careful individual titration is required. Accumulation may occur in susceptible patients, leading to a much prolonged elimination half-life.

Midazolam is usually used as an adjunct in the induction of anesthesia, short-term sedation, and also sedation on the intensive care unit.

• Diazepam

Diazepam has a longer half-life than midazolam (elimination half-life up to 60 h) and is usually administered as a bolus injection of 5–10 mg. It has active metabolites that have elimination half-lives of over 100 h.

It is usually used for the control of status epilepticus, short-term treatment of anxiety, and control of drug withdrawal reactions.

• Lorazepam

Despite a shorter elimination half-life than diazepam (8–25 h), Lorazepam has a longer duration of action due to less extensive distribution. Dosage is between 2–4 mg, administered intravenously, intramuscularly, or sublingually. Withdrawal effects of Lorazepam are severe if used regularly for an extended period.

It is used as an adjunct to anesthesia, for control of short-term anxiety, and also for the treatment of status epilepticus, where it is preferred to diazepam, because of its longer period of action.

Propofol

Propofol is a phenol derivative, and is presented as a white emulsion made up with soya oil, and egg phosphatide. The concentration may be 1% (most common) or 2% (used occasionally on the intensive care unit to limit lipid accumulation).

The mode of action remains unclear, although interaction with GABA and glycine inhibitory neurotransmitters may contribute to its effects.

It is used for:

• Induction of anesthesia
• Maintenance of anesthesia
• Short- and long-term sedation on the intensive care unit
• Treatment of status epilepticus
• As part of patient-controlled sedation techniques

Propofol is becoming increasingly popular as a means of sedation on the intensive care unit. The reason for this is that it is short acting, exhibits rapid offset, is metabolized in the liver to inactive metabolites, and has little long-term hangover effect. The elimination half-life is between 10 and 70 min.

However, it has significant negative inotropic effect, causes significant vasodilatation, and reduces cardiac output significantly. Its use in critically ill patients requires extreme care.

The dose for the induction of anesthesia is approximately 2 mg/kg, although this requires modification in the obese patients. Sedation is normally achieved with infusion rates between 1 and 10 mg/kg/h.

Barbiturates

This class of sedative agent is thought to act by depressing postsynaptic sensitivity to neurotransmitters, and reducing the presynaptic release of these transmitters. The reticular activating system is particularly sensitive to the action of barbiturates.

• Thiopentone

Thiopentone is the most commonly used barbiturate on the intensive care unit. It is generally used only in specific circumstances, such as:

– Induction of anesthesia, particularly for rapid sequence induction
– Brain protection and control of intracranial pressure
– Treatment of status epilepticus

However, thiopentone is used very rarely for general sedation on the intensive care unit. The main disadvantage to thiopentone is the exceptionally long duration of action when administered by infusion, and the elimination half-life of up to 22 h. It may also cause tissue necrosis if it extravasates, and thrombosis if injected intraarterially. It is metabolized in the liver, and the inactive metabolites are excreted in the urine.

Thiopentone is a negative inotropic agent, reducing cardiac output by up to 20%. It should be used with caution in the critically ill. A degree of bronchoconstriction may also occur. It should be avoided in porphyria.

It presented as a powder, which is made up to a 2.5% solution, which is significantly alkaline (pH10.5). The dose for the induction of anesthesia is 3–6 mg/kg, and for sedation, 1–5 mg/kg/h, titrated to the effect on either intracranial pressure or EEG.

Ketamine

Ketamine is a phencyclidine derivative, and acts as an NMDA receptor antagonist, reducing flux in the calcium ion channel. It also inhibits phencyclidine binding with the NMDA receptor, further reducing activity. It also has some opioid receptor agonism effects. It produces a state of dissociative anaesthesia, a useful combination of light sleep and analgesia.

It is usually presented as either 10 mg/ml, 50 mg/ml, or 100 mg/ml clear solutions.

Ketamine is used in anaesthesia, on intensive care, and also in A&E, as well as out-of-hospital situations. Its main uses are:

- Induction of anesthesia
- Analgesia, particularly in burns patients requiring frequent dressing changes
- Sedation
- Bronchodilator in the treatment of status asthmaticus

Ketamine is particularly useful in that cardiovascular and respiratory reflexes are well preserved, cardiac output and blood pressure maintained, and it induces significant bronchodilatation.

A disadvantage of the use of ketamine is the occurrence of hallucinations, delirium, and unpleasant dreams. These may be less frequent in the young and old. This effect may be reduced by the administration of benzodiazepines, opioids, and droperidol.

Increased salivation and postoperative nausea and vomiting may occur.

Ketamine is metabolized in the liver, to partially active metabolites, which are then excreted in the urine. It has an elimination half-life of 2.5 h.

The dose for the induction of anesthesia is 1–2 mg/kg intravenously. Continual sedation requires an infusion rate of 10–50 µg/kg/min. Analgesia may be attained by intramuscular injection of 2–4 mg/kg, or an infusion of 4 µg/kg/min. Ketamine may also be used as an agent in patient-controlled analgesia devices.

Due to its cardiovascular effects, Ketamine is widely used in the induction of patients who are hypotensive. However, it should be used with caution in patients with known coronary artery disease due to the tachycardia and increased myocardial oxygen consumption. It should not be used in hypertensive patients and those with existing cerebrovascular disease.

Ketamine has been shown to increase both intracranial pressure and cerebral metabolic rate. Ketamine and other NMDA receptor antagonists have however been shown to reduce the release of excitatory amino acids in Ischemic and traumatic brain injury. This effect may be offset by the changes in intracranial pressure and metabolic rate; Ketamine should therefore be used with caution in head injury patients.

Ketamine also induces a sympathetically mediated bronchodilatation making it an ideal agent in patients with reversible airways disease either alone or in combination with other agents. The use of Ketamine as an adjunctive analgesic has been shown to reduce opioid requirements acutely (Schultz et al 2003) and may also reduce the incidence of chronic pain syndromes.

Isoflurane

Gaseous agents are used rarely on the intensive care unit, because they require specialist equipment, such as vaporizers and gas scavenging. However, there are circumstances where agents, particularly isoflurane may be used.

Isoflurane is a halogenated hydrocarbon that is liquid at room temperature. It is stored in dark Color-coded bottles (purple), and a specific vaporizer is used to deliver the gas in a known percentage concentration.

The mechanism of action of general anesthetic agents remains somewhat unclear, but the action may involve the disruption of neurotransmitter release and action, both pre- and postsynaptically.

Isoflurane is used for:

- Induction and maintenance of general anesthesia
- Sedation on the intensive care unit, particularly in severe asthmatics
- As a component of "Isonox" for relief during childbirth, via a demand valve

An advantage of isoflurane is that excretion occurs via the lungs, with only 0.2% being metabolized in the liver. Accumulation is therefore not a problem.

However, isoflurane is a significant vasodilator, and a mild cardiac and respiratory depressant.

General anesthesia is maintained at a concentration between 0.5 and 2%. Sedation may be achieved at concentrations of 0.2–0.8%. Its use in obstetrics is limited to a maximum concentration of 0.2%.

Antipsychotics

This class covers a variety of agents used for the control of delirious, aggressive patients on the intensive care unit. They are very useful, but extensive use in large cumulative doses may cause permanent unwanted side effects in patients. They should therefore be used with caution.

- Haloperidol

A butyrophenone is available for oral, intravenous, or depot intramuscular use. Haloperidol exerts an antidopaminergic type 2 receptor blockade centrally, and also acts at the GABA receptor in the CNS.

It is used for:

- Sedation
- Reducing motor drive and aggression (neurolepsis)
- Antiemesis
- The treatment of schizophrenia and other psychoses

Haloperidol is extremely useful in controlling the delirious and aggressive patient on the intensive care unit, who may be a danger to themselves and others. It has minimal respiratory and cardiovascular effects, and a useful powerful antiemetic effect.

However, it has some significant side effects, the most significant of these being extrapyramidal effects such as dystonia, and tardive dyskinesia which may be irreversible. It may also cause a small degree of hypotension, especially in hypovolaemic patients.

Haloperidol is metabolized in the liver, excreted in the urine, and has an elimination half-life of over 10 h.

- Chlorpromazine

Chlorpromazine is a phenothiazine, available orally and intravenously.

It works in a similar manner to haloperidol, but in addition, has serotonergic, adrenergic, histaminergic, and cholinergic blocking effects, leading to a wider spectrum of action and side effects.

It is used for:

- Sedation and anxiolysis
- Neurolepsis
- Antiemesis
- Treatment of schizophrenia and other psychoses

It causes both cardiovascular and respiratory depression, and a decrease in salivation causing a dry mouth. Through its wide variety of pharmacological effects, it causes a further wide spectrum of side effects. Despite all these, it is surprisingly well tolerated and safe, but still may cause serious, possibly permanent extrapyramidal side effects. Chlorpromazine may cause contact sensitization among health workers and should be handled with care.

Chlorpromazine is metabolized by numerous pathways in the liver, to a wide variety of metabolites, some of which are active. Elimination half-life is about 30 h, and excretion is in the urine and faces.

Routes of administration include oral, intravenous, intramuscular, and rectal. Intravenous doses must be administered slowly to avoid hypotension.

- Olanzepine

Olanzepine is a newer "atypical" antipsychotic drug, which may have fewer extrapyramidal side effects. It may be used for:

- Sedation
- Control of mania and psychoses
- Neurolepsis

The main side effects are hypotension and glucose intolerance.

For Clonidine and Dexmedetomidine, see nonopioid analgesia section.

Opioids

Opioids, in addition to being the mainstay of analgesia on the intensive care unit, obviously have significant sedative properties, and are commonly used in conjunction with the sedative agents described above. These agents will be covered in detail in the section on analgesia.

Nonopioid Analgesia Within the Intensive Care Unit

Although opioids form the predominant part of analgesia provision within the intensive care unit, agents such as Paracetamol, Ketamine, Clonidine, and Dexmedetomidine as well as Tramadol and to a lesser extent, nonsteroidal anti-inflammatory agents have a role within the intensive care to provide multimodal analgesia minimizing opiate side effects and improving patient comfort.

Paracetamol (Acetaminophen)

Paracetamol has both analgesia and antipyretic effects, but has not been shown to have any useful anti-inflammatory properties. The precise mechanism of action of paracetamol is yet to be clearly established.

Oral Paracetamol is readily absorbed from the gastrointestinal tract with peak plasma concentrations occurring some 10–60 min after ingestion. Absorption via the rectal administration is variable.

At normal doses plasma protein binding is minimal. Metabolism is by liver enzymes and conjugation with glucuronide or sulfate. In adults, the glucuronide is the predominant metabolite and in infants and children sulfate. These metabolites are excreted in the urine with less than 5% excreted as unchanged paracetamol. The duration of action is 3–4 h, which may be prolonged in hepatic disease, the elderly, and the neonate.

Oral Paracetamol has a long history of being safe in pregnancy with small amounts crossing the placenta. Paracetamol also has a safe record in breast-feeding with less than 1% being excreted into breast milk. Paracetamol should be used with caution in patients with liver and renal impairment, although at normal doses of up to 4 g per day, it is neither nephrotoxic nor hepatotoxic.

Paracetamol is generally well tolerated, but in overdose, can result in severe liver damage and acute renal failure. In adults, hepatotoxicity may occur after the ingestion of 10–15 g, and a dose of 25 g is potentially fatal. Jaundice, hypoglycemia, metabolic acidosis, and bleeding may take at least three days to develop.

Recently, an intravenous preparation of paracetamol has become available (Perfalgan). It has a faster onset of action with an onset of pain relief within 10 min and peak analgesic effect in 1 h. Intravenous paracetamol (Perfalgan) achieves peak plasma doses approximately twice that of oral preparations at 30 μg/ml after about 15 min, but by 1 h, plasma concentrations are similar for oral and intravenous routes. The higher peak plasma concentration implies further caution when administering IV paracetamol to patients with significant hepatic impairment. There is minimal safety data or experience with intravenous paracetamol in pregnancy. No direct reproductive toxicity studies have been performed in animals with IV paracetamol; however, no signs of prenatal/postnatal toxicity were observed in rats with the prodrug proparacetamol at three times anticipated clinical doses.

For ketamine see Sedation section.

Clonidine

Clonidine is a very useful and probably underused drug on the intensive care unit.

It is an aniline derivative, and is a centrally acting antihypertensive drug. Clonidine (and Dexmedetomidine) is α_2 presynaptic receptor agonist, reducing the release of noradrenaline, reducing sympathetic tone, and lowering blood pressure. The analgesic effects are mediated by α_2 receptors in the dorsal horn of the spinal cord, as well as central actions. Spinal neuropeptides (such as substance P) are also reduced.

It uses are:

- Analgesia
- Adjunct to sedative agents
- Control of hypertension
- Treatment of drug withdrawal

It has minimal effects on respiratory rate. The reduction in blood pressure appears to be due to reduction in peripheral vasomotor tone, and perhaps to a lesser extent, a small degree of bradycardia. Cardiac output is reasonably well maintained. Clonidine may cause a degree of drowsiness, and a dry mouth.

Withdrawal of long-term clonidine requires care, as abrupt withdrawal may cause rebound hypertension and tachycardia. It is thought this may be due to the variable duration of central and peripheral effects.

Clonidine is metabolized partly in the liver, and both unmetabolized clonidine and its metabolites are excreted mostly in the urine. The elimination half-life is up to 24 h.

Dexmedetomidine

This is a drug similar to clonidine, in that it is a selective α_2 agonist, producing a degree of sedation, together with hypotension and analgesia. It is rarely used on the intensive care unit and is currently unlicensed in the UK. Dexmedetomidine has a shorter half-life and is a more potent α – agonist than Clonidine. Side effects include cardiac arrhythmias such as atrial fibrillation and bradycardia.

Tramadol

Tramadol is a centrally acting synthetic agent with opioid-like effects. The mechanisms of action of Tramadol have not been completely explained; however, in addition to its opioid effects, it also inhibits the reuptake of serotonin and noradrenaline. The opioid type effects come from its weak affinity to mu-opioid receptors and its prime metabolite mono-o-desmethyltramadol's high affinity to mu receptors. In animal models, the Tramadol metabolite is six times more potent at producing analgesia and has 200 times more affinity to mu receptors than Tramadol itself, although the contribution to analgesia in humans is unknown. The analgesic effects of Tramadol are only partially reversed by the opiate antagonist naloxone. The additional pharmacological actions of Tramadol contribute independently to the overall analgesic effect of Tramadol. There is a dose-dependent effect; however, plasma concentrations and analgesic effect vary widely with individuals. Apart from analgesia, Tramadol may produce similar side effects to opioids. However, it causes significantly less respiratory depression than morphine, and at therapeutic doses, it does not have significant clinical effect on heart rate, left ventricular function, or cardiac index.

Tramadol is predominantly metabolized by demethylation, glucuronidation, or sulphation in the liver; however, only the mono-o-desmethyltramadol is active. Its production is dependent on the cytochrome CYP450 isoenzyme CYP2D6 that displays considerable interpersonal differences. This may account for some of the differing analgesic effects of Tramadol between people. Approximately, 95% of Tramadol and its metabolites are renally excreted, with up to 35% of parent drug excreted in the elderly. Tramadol should be used in caution in those patients who have hepatic and renal impairment as they may show considerably lengthened plasma half-life.

Convulsions have been reported in those taking routine doses of Tramadol. It should be used with great caution in patients who have epilepsy or who are at risk of seizures. Tramadol should also be used with caution in those patients taking selective serotonin reuptake inhibitors to avoid serotonin syndrome.

Nonsteroidal Anti-Inflammatory Drugs

Nonsteroidal anti-inflammatory drugs (NSAIDS) act by reducing the production of prostaglandins by the inhibition of Cyclo-oxygenase enzymes (COX1 and COX2). Prostaglandins are involved in homeostatic functions and regulation of vascular tone and blood flow as well as the inflammatory process. The NSAIDS form a wide class of drugs with the newer agents generally being more COX2 specific. The inhibition of COX1 results in reduced prostaglandin synthesis and decreased mucus production. Newer COX2 selective inhibitors have been produced to decrease gastric ulceration. However, prostaglandins are involved with vascular endothelial function, vessel tone, and blood flow. Selective COX2 inhibition has not improved renal toxicity and may increase myocardial thrombotic events. As such, they should be used with caution in the critically ill patient.

Opiates in Critical Care

Introduction

Opiates are used extensively in the critical care for their primary effect of analgesia, but also in combination with other drugs for their sedative properties to aid mechanical ventilation. The specific choice of opiate depends on the drug pharmacodynamics, pharmacokinetics, route of administration, and physiological status of the critically ill patient.

The properties of different opiates in the critically ill patient can have profound effects on patient care (Table 3.1). Inadequate treatment can lead to pain and discomfort, producing patients who are difficult to manage on ventilators with the potential for long-term psychological effects. Pain can lead to endogenous catecholamine release and thus arrhythmias and hypertension. Excessive dosages can lead to hypotension, and decreased respiratory drive. The primary opiate in critical care is morphine. The piperidine derivatives such as fentanyl, alfentanil, and remifentanil are also used.

Pharmacodynamics

Clinically, there is very little difference between the actions of all the different opiates. They all act primarily as μ receptor agonists throughout the body, along with some action on κ and δ receptors.

Central Nervous System (CNS)

The main analgesic effects of opiates are mediated via the CNS. They also cause drowsiness and mental clouding, but little or no amnesia, and patients may also experience euphoria. Myosis also occurs, and combined with the drowsiness may make neurological examination difficult. Nausea and vomiting

TABLE 3.1. Effects of inappropriate analgesia with opiates on critically ill patients

Inadequate analgesia	Excess analgesia
Excess catecholamine release	Oversedation
Hemodynamic deterioration	Prolonged ventilation
Increased oxygen requirements	Increased risk of ventilator-
Increased catabolism	associated pneumonia
Agitation	Inability to communicate
	Hemodynamic instability

are unwanted side effects, which can be distressing if the patient is aware and unable to communicate, but often subside with prolonged treatment.

Respiratory depression results, even at low doses, from reduced responsiveness of the brainstem to CO_2, leading to the reduction in respiratory rate and tidal volume. This may have effects on patients weaning from ventilators and those with respiratory compromise. Antitussive properties of opiates, mediated via the medulla, may be beneficial in intubated patients, but potentially detrimental to those with retained secretions. High-dose fentanyl has been reported to cause severe muscle rigidity, believed to be caused by the stimulation of basal ganglia receptors, producing patients who are often very difficult to ventilate (wooden chest syndrome). Other CNS effects include altering the body temperature regulating center in the hypothalamus and reduction of the secretion of anterior pituitary hormones, the significance of which is unclear in critically ill patients.

Cardiovascular System

Opiates induce vasodilatation by a number of mechanisms including histamine release and inhibition of baroreceptor reflexes. Histamine release can be significant with morphine, but unusual with piperidine derivatives, making them the opiates of choice when there is cardiovascular instability.

Gastrointestinal Tract

Gastric motility is reduced even with small doses of opiates, and the peristaltic action of the small and large bowel is also reduced. This reduces gastric emptying, increases the incidence of esophageal reflex, and due to the increased time for water absorption, also leads to constipation.

Immune System

Exogenous opioids have been shown to have a multitude of actions on the immune system. These include altered T-cell function such as reduced cytotoxic K cell activity, altered graft vs host disease response, and depressed T-cell mediated antibody production by B-cells. Macrophage and monocyte function may also be affected. The clinical consequences of these immune system effects are still unclear.

Pharmacokinetics

In critically ill patients, the expected pharmacokinetic properties of opiates can be significantly altered due to the reduced liver and renal blood flow. Intrinsic organ function also fluctuates. Some opiates such as pethidine have seizure-inducing metabolites (norpethidine) that are usually cleared by the kidneys, and therefore, pethidine is rarely used in critical care. Opiates therefore require controlled titration of doses and careful monitoring. The pharmacokinetic properties of the various opioids are often more important in selecting an opiate, rather than pharmacodynamics (Table 3.2).

Route of Administration

In ITU, the intravenous route is the most reliable, either as single bolus injections, or more commonly by infusions. Some opiates such as fentanyl and alfentanil have short half-lives due to the redistribution of the drugs. During prolonged infusions, these opiates can accumulate in fat stores which then act as a reservoir, releasing the drug after infusions have been stopped.

Oral opiates are not commonly used, as critically ill patients have reduced intestinal blood flow and variable absorption, which may be exacerbated by abdominal surgery, ileus, or pancreatitis.

Subcutaneous routes are also unpredictable due to odema and variable subcutaneous blood flow due to low cardiac output or vasoconstriction. Transcutaneous fentanyl is constrained significantly by poor dose titration. The effects are delayed both in the onset of benefits and adverse effect.

Opiates are occasionally administered via the epidural route in combination with local anesthetics.

Morphine

Oral morphine is almost completely absorbed, but high first-pass metabolism by the liver means that the intravenous dose is one third of the oral dose.

Its clearance is dependent on liver blood flow and function; therefore, its half-life is prolonged in liver failure and in condition of reduced liver blood flow such as septic shock. It is glucuronidated by the liver to morphine-6-glucoronide (M6G) and morphine-3-glucoronide (M3G). M6G is a more potent analgesic than morphine, while M3G has antagonist properties at opiate receptors. These metabolites are cleared by the kidneys and the accumulation of M6G in renal failure can cause a significant prolongation of morphine action.

Fentanyl

Fentanyl is not given orally due to its very low bioavailability as a result of first-pass metabolism. It is 100 times more potent than morphine, as well as more lipid soluble with a large volume of distribution. These properties result in faster onset of effects and short half-life due to redistribution. However, during prolonged infusions, the half-life may be greatly increased. Clearance is primarily via the liver and dependant on liver perfusion and function, where it is metabolized to inactive metabolites. Impaired renal function has little effect on fentanyl clearance.

Alfentanil

Following boluses or prolonged infusions, alfentanil has shorter half-lives than fentanyl or morphine. Its clearance is also dependent on liver blood flow and function with no active metabolites and no significant change in clearance in renal failure. When given by infusion, the half-life of alfentanil is only slightly increased as it has lower lipid solubility than fentanyl, and therefore does not accumulate in fatty tissues.

Remifentanil

Remifentanil is a potent, selective μ agonist, which has rapid onset and a short half-life.

TABLE 3.2. Pharmacokinetic properties of opiates

	Morphine	Fentanyl	Alfentanil	Remifentanil
Equipotent dose	10 mg	100 µg	750 µg	10 µg
Relative lipid solubility	1	573	90	12
Volume of distribution (l/kg)	3.5	4	0.8	0.7
Terminal half-life (h)	3	3.5	1.6	0.2

However, it is metabolized by nonspecific tissue and blood esterases to inactive products, and so, elimination is not dependant on renal or liver function. This removes concerns of drug accumulation with prolonged infusions and allows for a more predictable elimination on discontinuation of the drug.

Conclusion

The choice of opiates in critically ill patients depends primarily on the clinical state of the patient and the degree of liver and renal impairment, as well as liver blood flow. As these can change, the dose of the selected opiate may need frequent adjustment and review to ensure adequate analgesia, while at the same time ensuring minimal unwanted effects and prevention of accumulation. Morphine is the gold standard and the most used opiate in intensive care due to its low cost and extensive experience with its effects; however, the piperidine derivatives have significant roles, especially in renal and liver failure.

References

Booth CM, Heyland DK, Paterson WG (2002) Gastrointestinal promotility drugs in the critical care setting: a systematic review of the evidence. Crit Care Med 30:1429.

Collier J (2004) Proton pump inhibitors for acute upper GI bleeding. DTB 42:41.

Cook DJ, Guyatt G, Marshall J et al (1998) A comparison of sucralfate and ranitidine for the prevention of upper gastrointestinal bleeding in patients requiring mechanical ventilation. N Engl J Med 338:791.

Heyland DK, Dhaliwal R, Drover JW et al (2003) Canadian clinical practice guidelines for nutrition support in mechanically ventilated, critically ill adult patients. J Parenter Enteral Nutr 27:355.

Mutlu GM, Mutlu EA, Factor P (2001) GI complications in patients receiving mechanical ventilation. Chest 119:1222.

Schultz MJ, de Jonge E, Kesecioglu J (2003) Selective decontamination of the digestive tract reduces mortality in critically ill patients. Crit Care 7:107.

Van der Spoel JI, Oudermans-van Straaten HM, Stoutenbeck CP et al (2001) Neostigmine resolves critical illness related colonic ileus in intensive care patients with multiple organ failure – a prospective, double blind, placebo controlled trial. Intensive Care Med 27:822.

Index